Achieving Competency-Based, Time-Variable Health Professions Education

Proceedings of a conference chaired by

Catherine R. Lucey, MD

Atlanta, Georgia | June 2017

Edited by Teri Larson

Published by Josiah Macy Jr. Foundation
44 East 64th Street, New York, NY 10065
www.macyfoundation.org

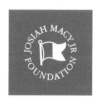

February 2018

CONTENTS

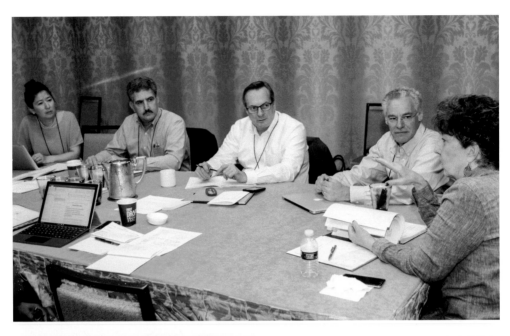

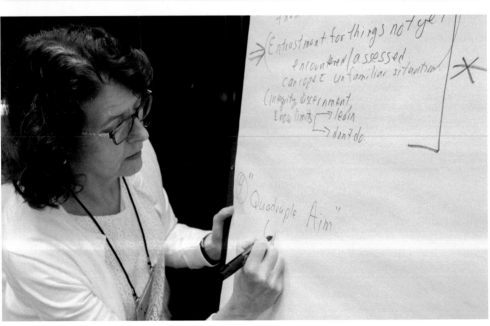

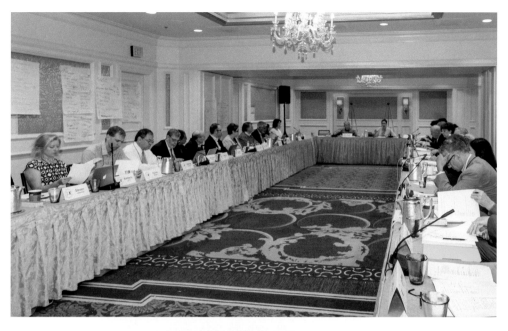

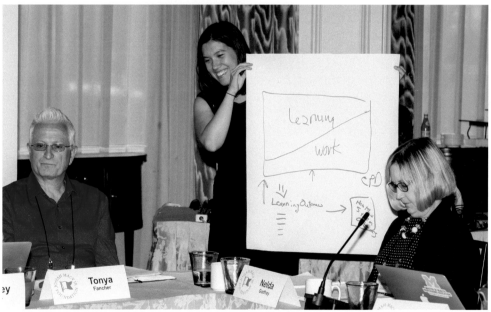

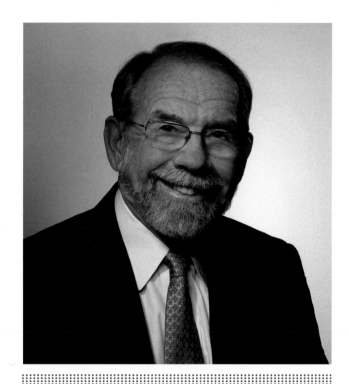

PREFACE

GEORGE E. THIBAULT, MD

The 2017 Macy Conference, *Achieving Competency-Based, Time-Variable Health Professions Education*, was perhaps the most ambitious of our conferences in the past decade because it addressed fundamental issues in the structure and pedagogy of all health professions education across the full continuum from beginning learners to experienced practitioners. We were emboldened to take on such an ambitious topic because advances in both theory and practice support a robust discussion of the pros and cons of radically changing our approach to educating the next generation of health professionals. We also felt an imperative to respond to the sense that our current educational enterprise is not fully meeting the needs of the patients we serve or of the learners we are educating.

The planning for a Macy Conference begins a full year before the conference, when we convene an interprofessional planning committee of educators and thought leaders to define the scope of the conference, draft a charge for the conferees, decide on commissioned papers and case studies, and draw up a list of potential conferees. We were blessed with a particularly experienced and insightful group chaired by Catherine Lucey, MD.

The conferees assembled in June in Atlanta, Georgia, were a diverse group of educators from nursing, medicine, pharmacy, and higher education with a mix of theoretical, clinical, measurement, and regulatory backgrounds. The two commissioned papers and three case studies formed the platform to begin the spirited and in-depth discussions that then went on for two and one-half days in plenary sessions and thematic breakout groups.

There were two major concepts that were the drivers of the discussion. The first concept is that of competency-based education. It was agreed that the competencies required for successful practice are derived from the needs of the patients and the public to be served. This realization changes the perspective of the processes of curriculum development and assessment. The second major concept is that of time as a resource in the educational process rather than a fixed endpoint. Embracing this concept would enable faculty and learners to allocate time as needed to accomplish the educational goal of competency. Such an approach would also require a change in learners' attitudes about the value of feedback, which would become the means by which learners progress to the next stage. All this will require developing a partnering relationship between faculty and learners, creating new and exciting roles for faculty and promoting a model for lifelong learning.

While becoming very excited about the enormous potential of this new model for health professions education, the conferees were also aware of the challenges in making such an ambitious paradigm shift. Consensus was reached on specific recommendations in five domains: (1) redesigning all elements of the learning environments; (2) creating a true continuum of education from novice to practitioner; (3) developing and implementing a robust assessment system; (4) developing and using enabling technologies; and (5) evaluating outcomes of learners, programs, and patients. There also was consensus that these innovations could not all be done at once, but that it is imperative that the process of change begin now. Early adopters can help pave the way for those that follow.

In the end, there was a unanimous feeling that these changes would be an essential part of creating a reformed health care system that better meets the needs of our patients. The conferees reaffirmed the importance of health professions education in improving the health of the public.

The success of a conference such as this depends upon many individuals. The conferees all gave of themselves unstintingly with energy, insight, and mutual respect. The planning committee facilitated the smooth running of the conference and the writing of the final report. All this was brilliantly led by Catherine Lucey as chair and staffed by Yasmine Legendre of the Macy Foundation.

This is both an exciting and an unsettling time in health care and health professions education. We all left the conference with a renewed sense of commitment to seize this moment to better align education with societal needs and real optimism that we have the tools and the will to do so.

George E. Thibault, MD

George E. Thibault, MD
President, Josiah Macy Jr. Foundation

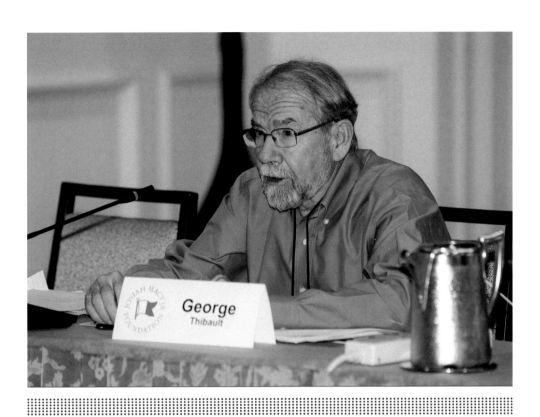

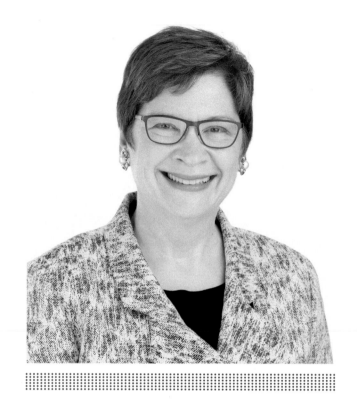

INTRODUCTION

CATHERINE R. LUCEY, MD
CONFERENCE CHAIR

The Institute for Healthcare Improvement Leadership Alliance has articulated its vision for the radical redesign of the health care system to achieve the following goals: care better than we've ever seen; health better than we've ever known; cost we can all afford—for every patient, every time.[1] When we achieve these goals, each patient who interacts with the health care system, whether for prevention, diagnosis, or treatment, will engage with professionals who are fully committed to, and measurably capable of, providing care that is safe, high-quality, equitable, efficient, effective, and patient-centered.[2]

Achieving this ideal health care delivery system begins with a carefully engineered educational continuum in which every health professional advances through the stages of formal education and into practice only when they have demonstrated mastery of all competencies needed to:

- provide compassionate and expert care to a diverse population of patients;

- function optimally within contemporary health care systems and interprofessional teams; and

- embark on a long career of lifelong learning and continuous assessment.

Our current time-bound, fragmented health professions educational systems do not yet fulfill this promise. Fortunately, advances have occurred in our pedagogical understanding of how health professionals attain expertise, alongside the tremendous biomedical advances of the past century. Application of educational theory to the complex workplace learning experiences of health professionals suggests that a revolutionary shift from course- and clerkship-based, time-bound education to competency-based, time-variable education is needed to bring us closer to the ideal system that meets the needs of our learners, our faculty, and, most importantly, our patients.[3,4]

Competency-based, time-variable (CBTV) education begins by designing educational programs with an explicit and relentless focus on the needs of patients and society for improved health and health care. In CBTV, health professions educational institutions continuously refine the competencies required of their graduates by monitoring evolving health care issues of patients and society; integrating advances in biomedical, social, and behavioral sciences; and leveraging opportunities provided by technological progress. Achieving this level of societal responsiveness requires a greater degree of adaptability in curricular planning and execution than our current educational institutions have demonstrated.[5,6]

CBTV education posits that the amount of responsibility and level of supervision assigned to each learner in the clinical environment must be determined by measuring competency, not by tabulating the number of weeks, months, or years spent in the program. The optimal design of CBTV programs would create a continuum of education across the years of formal training. Learners transition within and between programs when they can responsibly function with greater independence in their clinical care responsibilities and for their program of learning. This readiness for transition would be explicitly described using a set of demonstrable competencies in a variety of patient care experiences and assessed using a multimodal program of assessment. Faculty and learners alike would be aware of the requirements for competency development and together identify opportunities for the learner to be observed, assessed, and coached as they engage with different patients, in different contexts of care, with a variety of team members. Unlike the current model of education, assessment would not be a grade assigned at the end of a clerkship of predetermined length based on a general sense of the learner's ability. Instead, learners would be empowered to engage with faculty in a continuous process of goal-directed personal improvement. Faculty would use direct observation and feedback from team members and patients to support recurrent cycles of formative dialogue with learners about their strengths, weaknesses, and learning opportunities. Learners who meet competency goals prior to the usual end of a particular phase of education can either accelerate transition to the next stage of education or use additional time to deepen their competencies, engage in scholarly activities, or devote time to personal goals, such as family building.

Implementing CBTV education requires developing new programmatic and regulatory structures and models. Institutions that sponsor educational programs must support faculty development so that they are skilled in both goal-directed assessment and feedback. Compensation must be designed and time must be allotted during the workday for all members of the team to contribute input into the competency assessment of learners from all professions. Easy-to-use technology and tools must be deployed to collect data documenting learning and achievement of critical competencies. Academic institutions, licensing agencies, and certification boards must shift their requirements from time-based (credit hours, program length) to achievement-based parameters. Accreditors and regulators must redirect their attention to outcomes of education rather than to processes of education.

Proposed changes of this magnitude require careful analysis and planning. The 2017 Macy Foundation conference on achieving CBTV education set out to evaluate the evidence for embarking on this journey of pedagogical change for health professions education around the world. Experts in curriculum, assessment, professional identity formation, organizational change, and educational accreditation from medicine, nursing, and pharmacy came together to describe the opportunities of, outline the challenges associated with, identify unanswered questions about, and make specific recommendations to enabling a shift to a fully integrated system of CBTV health professions education. All agreed that the time has come to reshape health professions education of the 21st century to achieve our collective goal of ensuring that every patient has access to the type of health care professional that we would choose for someone we loved. We invite you to explore this topic with us and join us in this transformational movement.

Catherine R Lucey

Catherine R. Lucey, MD
Conference Chair

1. Feeley D, Berwick D, Duncan J, eds. *Institute for healthcare improvement leadership alliance prospectus year 4.* Boston, MA: Institute for Healthcare Improvement; 2017.
2. *Crossing the quality chasm.* 3. print. ed. Washington, D.C: National Academy Press; 2002.
3. Cooke M, Irby DM, O'Brien BC. *Educating physicians: A call for reform of medical school and residency.* San Francisco, CA: Jossey-Bass; 2010.
4. Frank JR, Snell LS, Cate OT, et al. Competency-based medical education: Theory to practice. *Med Teach.* 2010;32(8):638–645. doi: 10.3109/0142159X.2010.501190 [doi].
5. Lucey CR. Medical education: Part of the problem and part of the solution. *JAMA Intern Med.* 2013;173(17): 1639–1643.
6. Frenk J, Chen L, Bhutta ZA, et al. Health professionals for a new century : Education to strengthen health systems in an interdependent world. *Lancet.* 2010;376(9756):1923–1958.

CONFERENCE AGENDA

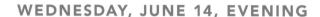

WEDNESDAY, JUNE 14, EVENING

3:00 – 6:00 pm	Registration
6:00 – 7:00 pm	Welcome Reception
7:00 – 9:30 pm	Dinner with Introduction of Conferees

THURSDAY, JUNE 15, MORNING

7:00 – 8:00 am   Breakfast

8:00 – 12:00 pm   **Session 1**

8:00 – 8:45 am   Brief introduction of participants and opening remarks
                    George Thibault, Catherine Lucey

8:15 – 8:50 am   Discussion of themes from commissioned paper
                    Time-Variable Training in Medicine: Insights Derived from the Literature and from Examples in Practice
                    Olle ten Cate
                    Moderators: Robert Blouin, Catherine Lucey

9:30 – 10:10 am   Discussion of themes from commissioned paper
                    Great Expectations: Competency-Based Medical Education from Reality to Vision
                    Damon Dagnone, Richard Reznick
                    Moderators: Debra Klamen, George Mejicano

10:10 – 10:30 am Break

10:30 – 10:55 am Discussion of themes from case study
                    The University of Wisconsin-Milwaukee Flexible Option for BSN Completion
                    Aaron Brower
                    Moderator: Juliann Sebastian

10:55 – 11:20 am	Discussion of themes from case study
	Describing the Journey and Lessons Learned: Implementing a Competency-Based and Time-Independent Undergraduate Medical Education Curriculum
	George Mejicano
	Moderator: Stephen Schoenbaum
11:20 – 11:45 am	Discussion of themes from case study
	Education in Pediatrics Across the Continuum (EPAC): Realizing the Dream of Time-Variable, Competency-Based Advancement in Medical Education
	Robert Englander
	Moderator: Carol Carraccio
11:45 – 12:00 pm	Charge to breakout groups

THURSDAY, JUNE 15, AFTERNOON

12:00 – 1:00 pm	Lunch
1:00 – 5:00 pm	**Session 2**
1:00 – 3:00 pm	Breakout Sessions
	Breakout 1
	Point/Counterpoint: Articulating the educational, economic, and philosophic case for CBTV education in formal health professions education programs. How will the naysayers respond?
	Moderators: Debra Klamen, Stephen Schoenbaum
	Breakout 2
	Educational enablers: the role of technology, faculty development, and other tools in CBTV education: What is needed? What do we already have?
	Moderator: Juliann Sebastian

Breakout 3

Challenging dominant paradigms: Re-designing educational systems, transitions, and accreditation strategies to facilitate CBTV education
Moderator: Carol Carraccio

Breakout 4

Building a bigger tent: What types of programmatic quick wins and incentives would convert CBTV skeptics into champions and followers?
Moderator: George Mejicano

Breakout 5

Identifying and mitigating unintended consequences: What are the risks to individual students, schools, and professions if we are misguided? Are negative consequences avoidable? Are they equally shared amongst all or do they disproportionately impact unique populations or specific professions?
Moderator: Robert Blouin

3:00 – 3:15 pm	Break
3:15 – 5:00 pm	Plenary Session
	Report out from Breakout Groups and general discussion of themes of the day to set agenda for the following day
	Catherine Lucey
5:00 pm	Adjourn

THURSDAY, JUNE 15, EVENING

6:30 – 9:00 pm	Reception & Dinner at the Carter Center

FRIDAY, JUNE 16, MORNING

7:00 – 8:00 am	Breakfast
8:00 – 12:00 pm	**Session 3**
8:00 – 8:30 am	Brief recap of Day 1 and Charge to Breakout Groups
	Catherine Lucey

8:30 – 11:30 am	Five Breakout Groups
	Breakout 1
	Assessment Strategies and Systems
	Moderator: George Mejicano
	Breakout 2
	Institutional Redesign: Admissions, Instruction, and Faculty Development
	Moderator: Debra Klamen
	Breakout 3
	Technology and Tools
	Moderator: Robert Blouin
	Breakout 4
	Regulatory and Other Systems: Accreditation, Licensing, the NRMP, the Boards
	Moderator: Carol Carraccio
	Breakout 5
	Individual, Program, and Societal Outcomes
	Moderators: Juliann Sebastian, Stephen Schoenbaum
11:30 – 12:00 pm	Group Photo

FRIDAY, JUNE 16, AFTERNOON

12:00 – 1:00 pm	Lunch
1:00 – 5:00 pm	**Session 4**
1:00 – 3:00 pm	Report out from Breakout Groups
	Moderator: Catherine Lucey
3:00 – 3:15 pm	Break
3:15 – 5:00 pm	Response to reports from Breakout Groups and identification of missing themes and recommendations
	Moderators: Catherine Lucey, George Thibault
5:00 pm	Adjourn

FRIDAY, JUNE 16, EVENING

6:30 – 9:30 pm   Reception & Dinner at Atlanta Grill

SATURDAY, JUNE 17, MORNING

7:00 – 8:00 am   Breakfast

8:00 – 11:45 am   **Session 5**
                      Conference Conclusions and Recommendations
                              George Thibault, Catherine Lucey
11:45 – 12:00 pm   Summary Remarks
                              George Thibault
12:00 pm   Adjourn

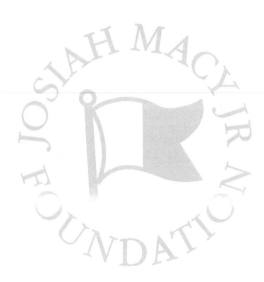

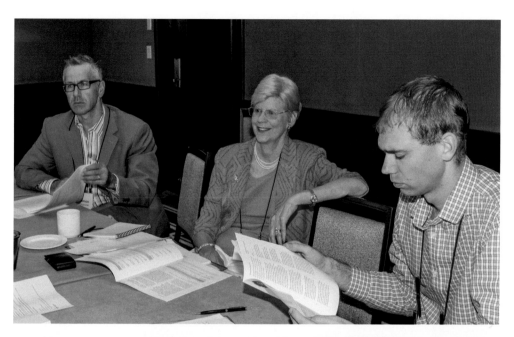

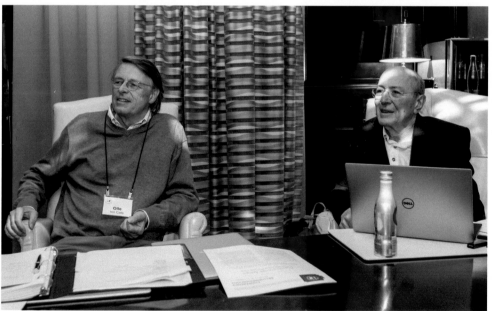

CONFERENCE PARTICIPANTS

Eva Aagaard, MD
Washington University School of Medicine

G. Rumay Alexander, EdD, RN
*The University of North Carolina
at Chapel Hill*

David L. Battinelli, MD
Hofstra Northwell School of Medicine

Anne R. Bavier, PhD, RN, FAAN
*University of Texas at Arlington College of
Nursing and Health Innovation*

Lisa M. Bellini, MD
*University of Pennsylvania Perelman School
of Medicine*

Robert A. Blouin, PharmD*
*The University of North Carolina
at Chapel Hill*

Barbara F. Brandt, PhD
*University of Minnesota
Academic Health Center*

Aaron Brower, PhD
University of Wisconsin-Extension

Carol L. Carraccio, MD, MA*
The American Board of Pediatrics

**Kathy Chappell,
PhD, RN, FNAP, FAAN**
American Nurses Credentialing Center

H. Carrie Chen, MD, PhD
*Georgetown University
School of Medicine*

Dorothy Curran, MD
University of Minnesota Medical School

J. Damon Dagnone, MD, FRCPC
*Queen's University
Faculty of Health Sciences*

Robert Englander, MD, MPH
University of Minnesota Medical School

K. Anders Ericsson, PhD
Florida State University

Jeffrey J. Evans, PhD
Purdue University

Tonya L. Fancher, MD, MPH
*University of California,
Davis School of Medicine*

**Nelda Godfrey,
PhD, ACNS-BC, RN, FAAN**
University of Kansas School of Nursing

Larry D. Gruppen, PhD
University of Michigan Medical School

Richard E. Hawkins, MD, FACP
American Medical Association

Eric S. Holmboe, MD
*Accreditation Council for
Graduate Medical Education*

Jan Jones-Schenk, DHSc, RN, NE-BC
Western Governors University

Adina L. Kalet, MD, MPH
NYU School of Medicine

Debra Klamen, MD, MHPE*
Southern Illinois University
School of Medicine

Steven A. Lieberman, MD
University of Texas Rio Grande Valley
School of Medicine

Kimberly D. Lomis, MD
Vanderbilt University Medical Center

Catherine R. Lucey, MD*
University of California,
San Francisco School of Medicine

Dylan Masters, MD
University of California,
San Francisco School of Medicine

George C. Mejicano, MD, MS*
Oregon Health & Science University
School of Medicine

Richard Reznick, MD
Queen's University
Faculty of Health Sciences

Denise V. Rodgers, MD
Rutgers Biomedical and Health Sciences

Stephen C. Schoenbaum, MD, MPH*
Josiah Macy Jr. Foundation

Daniel Schumacher, MD, MEd
Cincinnati Children's Hospital Medical Center

Juliann G. Sebastian, PhD, RN, FAAN*
University of Nebraska Medical Center

Olle (Th.J.) ten Cate, PhD
University Medical Center Utrecht

George E. Thibault, MD*
Josiah Macy Jr. Foundation

**Peter H. Vlasses,
PharmD, DSc (hon), FCCP**
Accreditation Council for Pharmacy
Education

Diane B. Wayne, MD
Northwestern University
Feinberg School of Medicine

Alison J. Whelan, MD
Association of American Medical Colleges

STAFF

Peter Goodwin, MBA
Josiah Macy Jr. Foundation

Yasmine R. Legendre, MPA
Josiah Macy Jr. Foundation

Ellen J. Witzkin
Josiah Macy Jr. Foundation

Teri Larson
Teri Larson Consulting

Katie Searle
EMCVenues

*Planning Committee Member

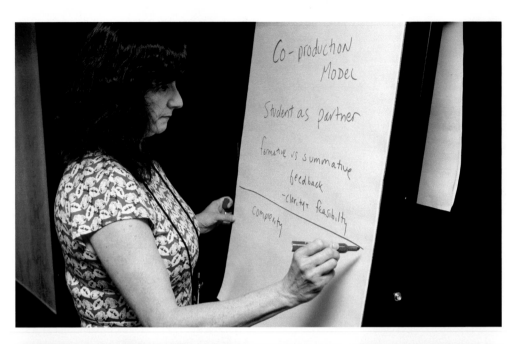

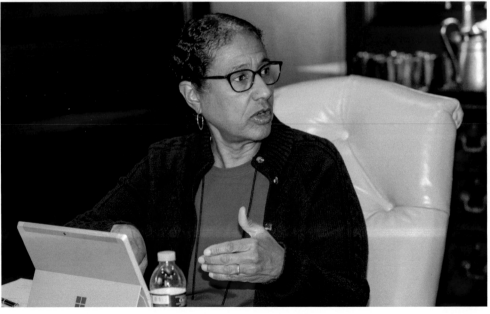

CONFERENCE CONCLUSIONS AND RECOMMENDATIONS

ACHIEVING COMPETENCY-BASED, TIME-VARIABLE HEALTH PROFESSIONS EDUCATION

Health professions education requires radical transformation to ensure delivery of high-quality health care in the 21st century. High-quality care begins with the education of our health professionals, who must be optimally prepared to meet the public's health care needs. Current approaches to health professions education are in evolution, as leaders of health professions education and healthcare delivery work to define the competencies needed to deliver care in our communities, implement new strategies for assessment, provide greater support for learner and practitioner well-being, and assure the public that the competence of their health care professionals remains superb across the continuum from formal education through decades of practice. Despite these efforts, however, health professions education is fragmented, time-bound, and too often disconnected from the practice of optimal pedagogies and existing health care challenges. To fulfill the social contract implicit in the provision of health care requires change that is more than evolutionary or incremental.

Now is the time for leaders of health professions education systems to partner closely with health systems executives, clinicians, researchers, accreditors, and our learners to revolutionize our educational approach, shifting it toward one of continuous learning, guided by the principles of competency-based, time-variable education.

Such a transformation will take time and will not be easy. Existing challenges in both health care delivery and health professions education are considerable. Despite almost two decades of concerns about the safety, quality, equity, accessibility, value, and patient-centeredness of health care in America, progress toward a system in which every patient receives the right care in the right place at the right time for the right cost has been slow. Challenges include the following:

- *Fragmented Care.* Patients with multiple and more complex chronic diseases are best served by health care that is continuous and integrated, but today's care remains too fragmented.

- *Slow Diffusion.* Advances in biomedical and behavioral science are potentially lifesaving, but their diffusion throughout the practice environment is slow and incomplete.

- *Disruptive Technology.* Electronic health records (EHRs) hold promise for improving the efficiency, safety, and precision of care, but their design clashes with existing systems of work, causing a tension that is contributing to a dangerous upswing in burnout among health professionals.

- *Ineffective Collaboration.* Health care professionals in many disciplines routinely earn advanced degrees and gain expertise in areas such as functional assessment, rehabilitation sciences, and therapeutic management equal to or surpassing physician competencies, yet true interprofessional collaborative practice that takes full advantage of all the health professions remains an aspiration rather than a reality in most health care systems.

Health professions education also faces many challenges, such as:

- *Information Explosion.* Substantial expansion of content relevant to the practice of medicine, pharmacy, nursing, and other health professions has led to concerns about curricula that are too dense at every stage of formal education.

- *Discontinuity in Education.* Optimal workplace learning requires stable, longitudinal assignments that enable students, residents, faculty, and patients to build relationships over time, but challenges such as monthly block rotations, work hours restrictions, shortened lengths of stay, and a shift from inpatient to outpatient care without a concomitant shift in educational venues have led to fragmentation and lack of continuity for both caring and learning.

- *Student Debt Burden.* The debt burdens of our students and trainees continue to escalate, causing significant stress and impacting career choices.

- *Faculty Burnout.* Faculty members, under intense pressure to maximize clinical productivity, have less time to spend teaching and assessing learners. Inherent in this time-pressured environment is a risk that lowering time spent on observation, assessment, and coaching of learners may fail to identify those who need more instruction and guidance to achieve satisfactory performance and limit opportunities for achieving excellence among all learners.

- *Assessment Challenges.* High-stakes decisions about advancement, retention, and graduation are made with persistent emphasis on multiple-choice exams, while robust assessments of critical competencies—such as clinical skills, communication, professionalism, and ethics—are not as widely used. Criteria for health professional certification and licensing need to be aligned with educational goals.

- *Marginalization of Patients.* Despite the importance of patient-centeredness as a critical element of health care quality, patients rarely have the opportunity to contribute to assessment of health professions students.

- *Challenges to Workforce Diversity.* The health professions workforce should reflect the diversity of the population served. More individualized approaches to learning that build upon what each learner brings to the educational environment will be a necessary component to diversifying the health professions workforce.

- *Inadequate Preparation for Transitions.* In medicine, pharmacy, and nursing, residency programs accepting new graduates and employers hiring newly licensed clinicians have raised concerns about inadequate training and deficiencies in critical competencies.

- *Inadequate Faculty Development.* Faculty members are committed to the concepts of remaining current and teaching new subject areas and skills, but many do not feel well-supported by existing systems for continuing education, professional development, and maintaining certification—which generally are not integrated into daily practice and are assumed to take place outside of the regular work day.

In response to these challenges, some health professions educators are championing a shift away from the traditional time-based educational system, in which learners spend a pre-determined amount of time in each phase of their health professions education, toward a competency-based, time-variable system, in which learners advance only after they have mastered specific concepts and skills. In fact, health professions educators within and outside the U.S. have taken critical foundational steps toward a competency-based, time-variable education system. We are now at an important inflection point; our current, predominantly time-fixed health professions education system must accelerate the transition to a competency-based, time-variable system.

In the U.S., the Accreditation Council for Graduate Medical Education (ACGME) launched the competency-based "Outcome Project" by describing the set of competency domains needed for physicians to better meet the health care needs of today's patients. ACGME's subsequent "Milestones" initiative, imbedded in the Next Accreditation System, attempted to define the developmental sequence of competency attainment and required programs to measure and report the progress of their residents. The Liaison Committee on Medical Education mandates that medical schools articulate graduation competencies and attest that their learners have met these competencies. Further, countries such as the Netherlands and Denmark have tested systematic efforts in competency-based education, and the College of Family Physicians of Canada has transformed all its residency programs to a competency-based model. Currently, the Royal College of Physicians and Surgeons of Canada has outlined a pathway to transition all its graduate medical education (GME) programs to a competency-based, time-variable system.

Further, since the early 1990s, the American Association of Colleges of Pharmacy through its Center for the Advancement of Pharmacy Education has developed and maintained educational outcomes for pharmacy students, the newest version of which has been incorporated by the Accreditation Council for Pharmacy Education into its PharmD program standards as expected competencies for new graduates.

The key targets are that, based on reliable assessments, pharmacy graduates are both "practice-ready" and "team-ready."

To review the current state of competency-based, time-variable health professions education—and to explore its potential to accelerate solutions to the challenges outlined above—the Josiah Macy Jr. Foundation hosted a conference on Achieving Competency-Based, Time-Variable Health Professions Education. The conference brought together 39 health professions educators in medicine, nursing, and pharmacy as well as experts in educational theory and reform, medical residents (learners), and education and residency program accreditors. They gathered in Atlanta and participated in two-and-a-half days of discussions leading to consensus around the recommendations presented in this report for designing and implementing competency-based, time-variable health professions education. By the end of the conference, the attendees had agreed upon the following vision for transformation of the American health professions education system:

> *With the achievement of competency-based, time-variable health professions education, we envision a health care system in which all learners and practitioners are actively engaged in their own education and continuing professional development to improve the health of the public. In this system, learners and faculty partner to co-produce learning, all practitioners are lifelong learners, and all health care environments place a high value on learning.*

This report provides an overview of the Macy conference on competency-based, time-variable education, including commissioned papers, themes, and recommendations.

CONFERENCE BACKGROUND

In a competency-based education system, learners progress by demonstrating the competencies they need to perform optimally as health professionals across the span of their careers—through the various stages of formal education, including transitions from one stage to the next, and into and throughout decades of practice. The desired competencies for optimal performance are based on what is needed to deliver health care of the highest quality and value to patients and their communities.

Competency-based education differs from traditional, time-based education in the way it views the continuum of learning and learner success, the nature of assessment, the roles and relationships of learners and faculty, and the design of educational experiences. Competency-based education approaches the entirety of a professional's career—from matriculation into health professions school to retirement—as part of the educational continuum. Learners are successful when they transition through different stages and different practice environments based not on their performance on an exam after spending a specific time in formal education, but on their ability to demonstrate measurable competence in the requisite set of behaviors needed to succeed at the next level or stage of performance.

When fully implemented, competency-based education provides assessment that is frequent (often daily), multi-modal, linked to explicitly defined performance goals, and based on observable behaviors. Learners in competency-based education systems are partners with faculty and patients in assessment; they know their competency targets and view assessment and feedback as welcome opportunities to receive critical coaching that allows them to progress toward their goals. In competency-based education, educational experiences are tailored to the assessed needs of the learner. In competency-based, time-variable training, time becomes a resource that learners use for their benefit. They have the freedom to dedicate additional time to work on mastery of a particularly challenging set of competencies; to use free time to pursue enrichment activities once competencies have been achieved; or to accelerate their transition to the next stage of training.

Many in education fear the term "time variability," believing that it would result in every student charting a totally independent course through their formal education, causing chaos within our institutions. But in competency-based education, time becomes a resource rather than a constraint. Time variability recognizes that competency acquisition is individual; it is a rare learner who simultaneously masters every competency needed to transition to the next stage of their career.

Learners who master some required competencies in less time than the total duration of their educational programs can shift their attention to more challenging competencies; move on to more advanced work; have time to engage in scholarly activities, such as research; or dedicate more time to family building and other extracurricular activities. Some learners may indeed be able to accelerate their transition into the next phase of their career. Conversely, learners who need additional time to master all requisite competencies are still viewed as successful once they meet the required competencies—in contrast to the stigma currently attached to failing to finish on time.

An important objective of competency-based, time-variable education is entrusting learners to provide care without supervision in relation to the professional competencies they have acquired. Faculty supervisors may formally entrust learners when they have demonstrated certain abilities and there is confidence that the learners have the capacity to perform equally well in situations that are similar but not identical. Entrustment derives from the construct, used in both medicine and pharmacy, of entrustable professional activities (EPAs), which are essential units of observable work that, in the aggregate, define each of the health professions. They provide the context for the competencies that professions have identified, and interestingly, many of these competencies are shared across health professions.

Successful assessment strategies are foundational to the conduct of a competency-based educational system. Many have assumed there is a single strategy that must be adopted to advance competency-based education. In fact, a number of different paradigms for assessment are compatible with a competency-based educational system, including EPAs, milestones, and the University of Wisconsin "Flex Option" competency sets (described in one of the papers commissioned for this conference). They share critical elements: each is designed to reflect the work that optimal-practicing health professionals must carry out at different stages of their careers; each is described using behavioral criterion; and each assesses the learner's knowledge application, skills, and habits of mind using direct observation as well as analysis of different types of evidence (e.g., written notes or multi-source feedback) submitted by learners.

Unfortunately, educational innovations targeting the achievement of a fully competency-based, time-variable system are constrained not only by traditional views of education but also by existing structures and systems, such as university registrar systems, licensing requirements, board certification standards, and accreditation systems that rely on credit hours and fixed durations of training as evidence of sufficient academic achievement. As an example, in medical education, the once-a-year matching structure and "all-in" rules of the National Residency Matching Program prevent learners from moving on to residency when they are ready.

Removing these and other barriers and facilitating the full implementation of competency-based, time-variable health professions education has the potential to result in the following benefits to society, educational institutions, and individual learners.

- Societal needs for high-quality care will be better met when health professionals' competencies are assessed and verified as they enter their profession, and are continuously assessed throughout their careers. This will advance our professions' abilities to fulfill our social contract.

- Learners' needs for rigorous, safe, and supportive educational environments will be better served by educational programs that encourage partnering with faculty in learning and assessment strategies while striving to achieve specific competencies, rather than competing with peers to outperform each other. Learning environments such as these have the potential to decrease toxic stress and burnout.

- Learners whose personal circumstances, abilities, and life goals allow or require them to master competencies at a different rate than their peers can do so without the fear of failing. Some learners may have the opportunity to advance earlier to the next stage of training, with potential economic and lifestyle benefits. At the same time, learners who otherwise might not consider entering the health professions (because of their non-typical learning styles, lack of educational opportunities, etc.) may find themselves drawn to competency-based, time-variable health professions education, which would permit the tailoring of the educational trajectory to their needs.

- Practicing health professionals, having been exposed to the benefits of assessment-driven learning during their formative educational/training years, will become skilled, lifelong learners who enthusiastically seek out specific assessment and learning experiences to continuously improve their competency throughout their careers.

- Interprofessional collaborative care will benefit from the establishment of explicit competencies and performance expectations relevant to all professions—such as the Interprofessional Education Collaborative's (IPEC) core competencies for interprofessional practice. This important work has the potential to increase the ability and opportunities of learners to work together to improve their performance and for faculty from all professions to supervise and coach learners from all professions.

- Educational institutions may find that participation in competency-based, time-variable educational programs creates more satisfaction for faculty as they see the benefits of assuming a role focused on the longitudinal support and coaching of young health professionals, rather than an episodic responsibility for judging students.

CONFERENCE PAPERS

Prior to the conference, participants read two commissioned papers and three case studies to ground them in the topic and prepare them for the work of the meeting.

The first paper, *Time-Variable Training in Medicine: Insights Derived from the Literature and Examples in Practice*, provided a thorough overview of time-variable medical training. The authors, Olle ten Cate, professor of medical education at University Medical Center in the Netherlands, and his colleagues Eugène Custers, Larry Gruppen, Lorelei Lingard, Pim Teunissen, and Jennifer Kogan, referred to such training as "related to the introduction of competency-based medical education" and "a shift from 'fixed time, variable outcomes' to 'fixed outcomes, variable time' as a desirable target for the future of medical training." They describe time in medical education as "already variable" because it differs around the world, with much more time flexibility built into the medical education models found in other countries. They also explain that there appears to be no research evidence to justify specific training lengths, and go on to describe reasons why time variability is now of interest to medical educators who are interested in better controlling the outcomes of training. The paper cites specific examples of successful programs employing this paradigm and describes several conceptual, theoretical, and practical aspects of time-variable training.

The second paper, *Great Expectations: Competency-Based Medical Education from Reality to Vision*, was authored by Damon Dagnone, associate professor of emergency medicine and faculty lead on competency-based postgraduate medical education, and his colleagues Denise Stockley, Leslie Flynn, and Richard Reznick at Canada's Queen's University. Based on the authors' experiences with converting the university's 29 residency programs to a competency-based, time-variable approach, it provided conferees with a blue-sky vision for the future of health professions training. It also explained the movement toward competency-based education taking place in medical education programs around the world, describing it as a response to more traditional educational models that assume learner competence based on the amount of time spent on task.

Each of the three case studies focused on efforts to design and implement a competency-based, time-variable education program. One case study outlined the University of Wisconsin (UW) Flexible Option for BSN Completion offered through UW-Milwaukee. Another described the journey and lessons learned during the implementation of a competency-based and time-independent undergraduate medical education curriculum at Oregon Health & Science University School of Medicine. A third detailed the competency-based, time-variable Education in Pediatrics Across the Continuum (EPAC) program, which is supported by the Association of American Medical Colleges and the Macy Foundation in four medical schools that have established pilot programs for competency-based, time-variable advancement in undergraduate and graduate education in pediatrics.

CONFERENCE THEMES

During conference discussions, several important themes surfaced repeatedly as conferees processed insights and lessons gleaned from the papers and case studies and began honing in on recommendations.

1. Health professions education systems, the clinical practice system in which learning occurs, and the educators and learners who participate in the system all have a responsibility to patients to continuously improve and evolve. A learning continuum that views time as a resource to be optimized rather than as a constraint, and that ensures mastery of well-defined competencies, supports this goal. Further, when health professions education is learner-centered and outcomes-oriented in this way, it becomes a more supportive environment for teaching interprofessional, patient-centered care.

2. Principles of competency-based, time-variable education must be applied across all the health professions and across the whole continuum

of education throughout the careers of health professionals. Viewing learning as a continuous process that spans different settings and phases reduces the pressure to master everything in any individual phase. It also has the potential to facilitate earlier differentiation for learners who know their preferred career trajectory and who wish to tailor their educational experience to optimize preparation for that career. Learning at every stage can build on learning from the previous stage, ensuring that the learner masters the competencies necessary to be successful.

3. A learner-engaged, robust assessment strategy must underpin the competency-based, time-variable approach to health professions education. The learner in this transformed educational system must be an active and engaged partner in ongoing and frequent assessment experiences rather than a passive recipient of a grade at the end of a rotation. The assessment strategy must target all relevant competencies using multiple modalities (including direct observation and input from patients and other team members).

4. Required competencies must be broad and developmentally based. They must encompass the requisite knowledge, skills, behaviors, and attitudes expected of health professionals at each stage of their development within their specific profession and discipline. It was noted that even with the most comprehensive competency framework, some aspects of professional development are challenging to measure, particularly professional identity formation. Conferees acknowledged that maturation time in a supportive educational environment—beyond what is needed to master competencies—may be required for learners to fully internalize their identities as professionals.

5. Full implementation of a competency-based, time-variable educational strategy will require health professions schools and training sites to develop a strategy to manage such a major change. All stakeholders (learners, faculty, administrators, staff, regulators, and communities served) must be included in the process. Much attention must be paid to faculty who will need to take on new roles and acquire new skills. Throughout this process, attention must be paid to the concerns of learners and faculty about possible adverse or unintended consequences of these changes.

6. Conferees agreed that the educational paradigm shift should be interprofessional and should include interprofessional competencies, such as those developed by IPEC. It is important for the development of all health professionals that both teaching and assessment are interprofessional. Currently, interprofessional, competency-based, time-variable education is uncharted territory. Developing it requires building relationships and mastering team-focused attributes, such as trust, communication, and collaboration.

When advocating for a major paradigm shift in complex systems, however, it also is necessary to consider scale. While one of the papers prepared for the conference describes the ambitious effort at Canada's Queen's University to introduce competency-based education simultaneously into the medical school's 29 residency programs, the other papers described efforts with a more limited scope. The conferees, while firmly supportive of competency-based, time-variable education as a goal, recognize that it will take different forms at different institutions and so encourage experimentation and customization. In fact, there is an immediate and ongoing need for research related to all facets of the concept, from design and implementation to learner assessment and program evaluation. Such research will better help us understand both the strengths and limitations of the concept.

MEASURES FOR SUCCESS

Although pilot programs in competency-based, time-variable education have confirmed the potential of this approach, moving forward requires institutions capable of implementing and studying its impact, describing the conditions under which it is both successful and unsuccessful, and contributing to the success of other institutions. The Macy conferees identified several conditions for success that will need to be met by institutions undertaking this paradigm shift. These include:

- Committed institutional leadership and an explicit plan for organizational change management,

- Agreed upon program outcomes and measures of success for each profession,

- A program of assessment tied to these outcomes,

- A well-thought-out implementation strategy,

- A willingness to break down barriers across the professions and across the continuum of education, and

- A willingness to work with regulators to remove barriers.

Certainly, some institutions engaged in educating the health care workforce are primed and eager to implement competency-based, time-variable health professions education. Other institutions, however, are not likely to be early adopters of this educational model. Our hope is that regardless of whether an institution adopts the model, all institutions will benefit from the research and implementation science work that their peer institutions do in pursuit of understanding how competency-based, time-variable training can contribute to optimal lifelong knowledge, skills, and habits of mind among health professionals.

Based on the commissioned papers and case studies, the rich plenary and breakout group discussions, and the experience of the conferees, consensus was reached around the following recommendations. The conferees felt all the recommendations were equally important and needed to be enacted together, not sequentially. They also felt an urgency to undertake this paradigm shift immediately so as not to further delay societal benefits.

CONFERENCE RECOMMENDATIONS

Recommendation I: System Redesign

Curricula, learning environments, and faculty development require systematic redesign to achieve a successful competency-based, time-variable health professions education system.

Competency-based assessment must be adopted as the strategy by which all health professionals navigate their formal education, transition into advanced training and then into practice, and demonstrate their continued effectiveness across the lifespan of their careers. Realization of the potential of competency-based, time-variable education requires integration of the work of the numerous distinct organizations currently charged with the conduct and oversight of multiple stages of health care professionals' education and assessment and will require significant system redesign. Leaders, accreditors, and licensors of organizations that provide health professions education and health care must immediately develop the necessary infrastructures to facilitate adoption of and to support the success of competency-based, time-variable education for learners across the continuum of health care careers, from students through practicing professionals.

Actionable Recommendations

1. National consortia representing health professions educators, health care delivery systems, academic health centers, community-based health systems and practices, practicing health professionals, learners, and patients must continuously identify critical population health and health care delivery goals and establish or update health professional competencies that ensure the health professions workforce is capable of successfully addressing contemporary health issues.

2. Each profession and its regulatory bodies must define readiness for learner transitions across the educational continuum and into practice by describing the comprehensive set of demonstrable competencies that indicate a learner is ready to advance, rather than by dictating the time the learner must spend in a given educational stage. Institutions must be held accountable for the decisions they make to allow learners to advance from highly structured and tightly supervised environments (such as medical, pharmacy, and nursing schools) to more flexible environments in which supervision is less direct (such as residency training programs) to fully autonomous practice.

3. Leaders of health professions education programs should evaluate and redesign, where necessary, curricula, programs, and methods of assessment to prepare their learners to demonstrate the competencies they need to contribute to the workforce that achieves the established health care goals. Learning activities and assessment strategies should be sequenced by the desired outcomes at each phase of education, training, and practice. Milestones of competency acquisition should be delineated to allow learners and faculty to understand the developmental trajectory expected of learners as they work to be entrusted with progressively more challenging work with less intensive supervision. This will require change

management strategies involving all stakeholders in the educational process.

4. Health professions education programs must invest in expertise to support competency-based, time-variable curricula. Experts in curriculum and assessment must engage teams to manage the design, implementation, evaluation, and continuous improvement of new learning and assessment strategies. These teams must involve or seek ongoing input from multiple stakeholders, such as patients, learners, and faculty as well as from experts in interprofessional collaborative care, data science, technology, and organizational change. Experts in faculty development must be charged with supporting faculty as they master new roles (such as coaching) and use new tools (such as performance dashboards) to support their learners. Experts in instructional design, technology-enhanced education and library sciences should collaborate on strategies and systems for optimizing learning throughout the entire continuum. They should be charged with developing and curating learning objects (videos, patient cases, teaching tools, simulation models, etc.) so that students, residents, and practicing professionals can access learning tools when they are ready to learn rather than wait until a formal course is offered. Technology systems for collecting longitudinal data about student performance and competency attainment across the continuum, such as electronic portfolios (e-portfolios), will be needed (see Recommendation IV).

5. Academic institutions should redesign promotion and tenure systems as well as faculty compensation models that recognize and reward faculty whose scholarly work focuses on the design, implementation, and continuous improvement of competency-based, time-variable education. Faculty compensation models and work schedules for health care professionals who supervise learners in the clinical environment should reflect the time needed to observe, coach, assess, and support learners in the competency-based, time-variable model.

6. Health care institutions should design health care environments to support workplace learning and assessment by all members of the team as part of the normal workflow. These environments should include interprofessional practitioners and learners within an aligned competency-based framework through all stages of learning, including continuing

professional development. Time must be built into the workflow to enable multi-directional, interprofessional assessment feedback to learners and practicing professionals.

Recommendation II: Creating a Continuum of Education, Training, and Practice

Institutions responsible for health professions education and health care delivery as well as those who lead, learn, and work within them should embrace the view of health professions education as a learning continuum that spans formal education, clinical training, and professional practice.

To maximize the effectiveness and the efficiency of competency-based education, learners must be able to move from one phase of learning to the next, building on and reinforcing what came before as well as laying the foundation for what comes next. It is incumbent upon the systems in which health professionals learn, train, and practice to ensure that the transitions between phases and throughout a career are as seamless as possible. Continuity of learning experiences not only leads to optimized learning but also provides the opportunity to align educational outcomes with the health needs of the populations served. The benefits of competency-based education can only be realized when transitions between phases are based on attainment of competencies rather than time.

Actionable Recommendations

1. Accreditors, regulators, certifiers, and educators in each health profession should examine and revise time-based policies governing transition points between phases of education. The internal programmatic logistics of time variability, in which a learner progresses from one phase to the next phase of structured training at an individual pace, may be daunting. This is especially true when education and service are inextricably linked. Other barriers that must be mitigated include inflexible financial models that are time bound (e.g. financial aid, tuition, stipends, etc.) and current National Resident Matching Program rules for physicians, which require a fixed time and process for transition from undergraduate to graduate medical education and from residency to fellowship.

    Experiments with an alternative "transition-to-practice phase" are underway at Queen's University in Ontario and may allow a more logistically manageable model of time variability. In this environment, learners who have been entrusted to perform the required activities of their profession enter a transition phase, which ends at the previously scheduled training completion date. During the transition phase, certification or licensing examinations are held. Learners are allowed to become certified and credentialed, increasing their clinical responsibilities as well as their supervisory and teaching roles. Patients and junior learners benefit from their experiences, the institution realizes greater reimbursements, and those in the transition-to-practice phase benefit from remote supervision in a supportive environment before facing autonomous practice.

2. Learners should be active navigators of the education, training, and practice continuum, with institutional support to develop the skill sets needed to follow their individual career roadmap. In a competency-based, time-variable educational environment, learners are expected and empowered to own their learning and assessment and to be actively involved and invested in working to ensure that faculty in current and subsequent learning experiences or environments are aware of and invested in helping them to build on strengths and fill identified gaps. Alignment along the continuum provides the opportunity to use many of the same assessment tools and strategies throughout all phases, providing each learner with a trajectory of performance over time.

3. Health professions education programs and the clinical institutions in which learners train should prioritize continuity between faculty and learners within each educational phase as a guiding principle critical to professional formation. Longitudinal assignment of students to faculty and clinical sites provides the time learners need to practice and fosters the trust in their supervisors that learners need to seek and accept assessment and coaching. The longitudinal, integrated clerkship (LIC) for medical students is one example of such an experience. LICs engage learners in prolonged clinical learning experiences organized around the principle of continuity with patients as well as faculty. Nursing and pharmacy students who participate in immersive clinical experiences over a period of time are likely to see similar advantages with assessment and coaching. Longitudinal coaching relationships may provide an alternative strategy for continuity. The coaching role is one in which faculty work frequently with a group

of students across their formal educational program to provide ongoing observation, formative assessment, and advice to learners to support their competency development. Coaches may collect and incorporate data about their learners from other health professionals (e.g., supervisors of the student during a clerkship) to support accurate assessments.

4. Leaders of health professions education and their accrediting agencies should develop and implement an ethical and transparent governance system for sharing learner performance data that supports the development of learners and the safety of patients. Data sharing on individual performance promotes seamless educational transitions to help learners optimize their learning and supports appropriate decisions about supervision to safeguard the quality of patient care. To earn and maintain the public trust, the education and health care systems must be transparent with regards to the data they collect on the performance of their learners, the level of evidence used by faculty and program leaders to determine learner progression, the information provided to future employers about health professions students and trainees, and the clinical outcomes associated with learners when they are engaged in clinical practice. There should be a priori agreement between the learner and the oversight body on the core nature of the information that will be transmitted.

5. Licensing bodies should collaborate with certification boards to streamline processes for initial licensing, re-entry, and re-training, and facilitate the continuous and meaningful assessment of ongoing learning and improvement over a health professional's career. Practice is a time for informal transitions, career evolution, and continuous professional development. Strengths and gaps from the prior phase should set the initial agenda for this phase. Maintenance of needed knowledge and skills as well as acquisition and application of new knowledge and skills will need to be addressed throughout the span of a professional career. Standardizing licensure processes and repurposing learning activities and their documentation will streamline the burden for learners, educators, and accreditors.

6. Federal and philanthropic dollars should be allocated to support the design and conduct of implementation studies that track a cohort of learners from various health disciplines through phases of education and training into

practice to determine the effects of transmitting core information about the learner from one phase to the next. Such studies may take a qualitative approach that examine 1) the impact on a learner's performance trajectory and self-efficacy; 2) how a program responds to the information received to benefit the learner; and 3) any unintended consequences.

Recommendation III: Implement a Robust Program of Assessment

Leaders in health professions schools and their health care system partners should champion, develop, and implement a program of assessment that supports competency-based, time-variable training and explicitly links educational programs to improved health care outcomes.

The assessment of students, trainees, and clinicians in practice should occur in a reliable, transparent manner and the tools and processes used to determine learner competence should be sound. Moreover, the program of assessment should be feasible, valid, reliable, dynamic, and acceptable to all stakeholders. Continuous improvement of the program of assessment requires analysis of data obtained during assessment activities across the career of health care professionals in relation to care that they deliver and health care outcomes of the systems in which they work.

Actionable Recommendations

1. Students, trainees, and clinicians in practice should embrace a systematic approach to assessment that aligns with desired outcomes from both the educational system and the clinical delivery system. Opportunities for learning should align with these desired outcomes so that the health care system is a partner in the educational mission. The program of assessment should incorporate rigorous methods along with valid and reliable tools that provide longitudinal, quantitative, and qualitative data related to learners' development and progression. Whenever possible, metadata from learning management systems and EHRs should be incorporated. For example, demographic data about patient mix, different diagnoses encountered, preventive services offered, and average patient length of stay on different rotations could be used to guide curricular changes, help determine whether a set number of encounters are needed to determine competence,

and demonstrate the value that learners contribute in the health care delivery system.

2. Leaders in health professions education should ensure that assessment is optimally supported. This should entail fostering the development of a subset of faculty with specialized knowledge and skills related to competency-based, time-variable learning and assessment. Faculty expertise will be required in multiple roles, such as academic coaching and direct observation, together with the provision of meaningful, daily feedback in clinical settings. Faculty with skills in new areas, such as interpreting performance dashboards containing information from multiple sources and determining readiness for entrustment, will also be needed. These dashboards should contain longitudinal data about a learner's progression toward pre-determined educational outcomes.

3. Leaders in health professions education must ensure that multi-modal, longitudinal performance data are collected and tracked to monitor trends as learners progress along performance trajectories through a variety of classroom, simulation, and practice settings. The focus of assessment must shift toward frequent formative assessments for learning that support learners as they prepare for more formal summative assessments of learning. Performance dashboards and learning outcomes should be accessible to students, trainees, clinicians in practice, coaches, and instructors to help customize learning. The need for additional time for a given learner to master a set of competencies should be viewed as a normal part of the process rather than an indication of failure. Learner assessment should always be competency-driven and criterion-based. Traditional grading scales should be eliminated as they may foster among learners the appearance rather than the achievement of competence, as well as unhealthy competition, and may contribute to stress and burnout among learners at all levels.

4. Students, trainees, and health care professionals should take active rather than passive roles in their own learning (i.e., co-produce). Engaged learners willingly take on their professional responsibility to seek assessment that will improve their competence in delivering care in a compassionate and competent manner. Learners across the health professions and along the continuum should actively seek opportunities for guided reflection

(e.g., with a mentor) to assess their own performance dashboards, obtain feedback, participate in deliberate practice, and co-produce plans to learn. Learners must accept that a commitment to high-quality patient care means that advancement can only occur once they demonstrate sufficient competency, regardless of the time they have spent on an activity. Conversely, once a learning outcome, competency set, or entrustment is achieved, learners must be allowed to use acquired skills to consolidate learning and further develop their abilities.

5. Leaders in health professions education and faculty should commit to program evaluation using strategies based in implementation science and continuous quality improvement to monitor the effectiveness of the program of assessment, including the quality of learners' performance data. Transparent and defensible data about individuals, interprofessional teams, and the program of assessment itself should be used to inform decisions about curricular architecture, individualized learning plans, and learner progression.

6. Leaders in health professions education should study the effectiveness and outcomes of programs of assessment and disseminate their findings to the broader health professions community. Specific areas of research related to assessment of learners in competency-based, time-variable health professions education should include the following: identifying important characteristics (of individual learners, of interprofessional teams and cohorts, of faculty and coaching approaches, etc.) that affect learner progression; examining how educational program design (flexibility, time variability, interprofessional collaboration, support mechanisms, assessment models, etc.) affects learner and patient outcomes; and clarifying the costs associated with implementing a robust program of assessment.

Recommendation IV: Enabling Technologies

Health professions education and health care delivery institutions should develop and use enabling technologies in the implementation of competency-based, time-variable education throughout the professional education continuum of the practitioner.

To successfully implement a competency-based, time-variable health professions education or training initiative, it will be essential to use existing and create new technological systems, platforms, and tools geared toward a different kind of learner-educator relationship and an environment of continuous, frequent, longitudinal assessment. New technologies will need to interface with EHR systems to facilitate both learning and assessment. These technologies must address new approaches toward rapid, mobile, seamless tools that support administrative processes (e.g., student matriculation, tracking student assessment, predictive analytics, and communities of learning) and instructional needs (e.g., digital information and knowledge acquisition, enriched experiential augmentation through holographic manikin simulation and virtual reality, and telemedicine technologies). In addition, the development of transportable e-portfolios to support lifelong, competency-based learning will be necessary as learners assume active responsibility for their own learning.

Actionable Recommendations

1. Competency-based, time-variable health professions learning environments will require new and enhanced technologies and systems, both administrative and instructional. Administrative technologies will be needed to facilitate the management and tracking of a more complex student-learning experience that includes admission, registration, graduation, and transition tracking throughout the learner's professional career. These technologies must be capable of supporting documentation of academic progress for learners who will not be matriculating through a traditional semester-based academic structure. Institutions will need to move toward a more flexible accounting system that will recognize the diminished role of the credit hour and normative grading for tracking student progression. New transcript models will need to be developed to document competency acquisition rather than course hours and grades. Creating technologies and software solutions that will support student learners and educators throughout their transitions will be essential, particularly to support real-time student and resident development and assessment.

2. The creation and implementation of new instructional technologies will become increasingly important to support the learner in a competency-based, time-variable curriculum. Educational technologies should make curriculum and learning assets continuously available to learners to facilitate flexible pacing toward mastery. Tools that support continuous learning

and just-in-time assessment and feedback will need to be more flexible, accessible, and easier to navigate if they are to enable student learning in a new, more complex environment. These technologies will be needed to support a wide range of instructional objectives including, but not limited to, the following:

- creation and implementation of mobile software to support and enrich foundational knowledge acquisition;

- development of holographic manikin simulation and high-fidelity virtual reality technology to accelerate experiential learning; and

- incorporation of distance education and telehealth strategies to facilitate didactic and experiential learning by professionals enrolled in formal educational programs and engaged in practice-based learning, regardless of their location.

3. Health professions educational institutions should develop strategic partnerships and collaborations in the form of consortia that will facilitate the creation and sharing of novel and interoperable platforms and tools to aggregate relevant performance data from multiple sources on individuals, groups of individuals, and programs. There is a paucity of commercially available solutions to support competency-based, time-variable curricula. Strong commitment from institutional leadership is essential to create demand at scale to generate commitment from vendors and others to develop flexible, responsive technology that supports competency-based, time-variable education. These tools need to be developed in a manner to amplify interprofessional activities of learners and educators while maintaining the highest level of data stewardship. Current challenges to data stewardship include compatibility and interoperability between solutions and data, the limitations of privacy laws, ethical concerns around data sharing, and discoverability of data. Data stewardship must include flexible means for stakeholders to opt-in and opt-out of data sharing, such as longitudinal tracking of learners, faculty, and patient records.

4. Consortia of health professions educators and institutions, technology experts, and data scientists should create, develop, and deploy rapid, real-time assessment tools using hand-held and mobile technologies. Mobile

technologies can provide learners with immediate assessment feedback and educators with rapid and efficient mechanisms to track and evaluate learner progress throughout the learning continuum. These tools must be integrated with data analytic systems that will enable a continuous assessment of learners as they progress through the various transitions of clinical learning and practice environments within urban and rural settings. Further, these robust tools must enable learners to connect continuously, including within interprofessional practice environments.

5. Academic institutions will need to encourage and support educational scholars and data scientists to investigate the use of data analytics to assist in planning educational trajectories for different students. It is essential to capture critical information and data from students and educators to support learners and educators throughout the learning process. From the point of admission, learners' data can be used to anticipate opportunities to enhance learning and mitigate challenges to optimize performance. These analytics will be necessary to individualize the educational experiences of our learners.

6. Digital learning communities should be developed to support learners and educators. These digital homes will facilitate the sharing of best practices associated with learners and educators within and among the health professions to accelerate learning within the didactic and experiential settings. The creation and sharing of learning platforms, including e-portfolios to support longitudinal training throughout the learner's lifetime, will facilitate integrated, interprofessional training.

Recommendation V: Outcomes Evaluation

Competency-based, time-variable health professions education programs should be designed, implemented, and evaluated in relation to preparing their graduates to advance important societal goals, including improved patient care and improved practitioner performance and satisfaction.

Competency-based, time-variable health professions education is a transformational approach to both education and health care. With a relentless focus on achieving desired care outcomes, each stage of a health care professional's education, training, and career is linked by a set of competencies aligned across the continuum. The continuity of focus catalyzes the development of a cycle of continuous improvement, where educational outcomes are linked to and influenced by societal goals for health care outcomes. Achieving this will require all to commit to a guiding principle of transparency, establishing patient registries for learners as well as practitioners, and multi-directional exchange of outcomes data to ensure accountability of the system in meeting both educational and health care outcome goals. Learners should be able to review their performance on all types of assessment instruments. Faculty should be able to review feedback on their instructional effectiveness as well as on how learners they assessed performed at the next level of training and/or in practice. Leaders in health professions education should provide accurate information to those who work with learners following a transition, such as from graduation to residency. Employers should provide data back to the educational programs that participated in the training of their employees.

Actionable Recommendations

1. Leaders in competency-based, time-variable health professions education programs should employ rigorous program evaluation models that track individual and aggregate competency development trajectories and outcomes. These models must include data on learner performance before and after critical transitions between institutions and phases of education and career to measure the effectiveness of a program's system of learning and assessment.

2. Health professions education programs should track educational metrics and associated outcomes of individual learners that reflect the essential competencies needed to meet societal needs for high-quality health care. This tracking includes standard outcomes measures such as licensing, board certification, and maintenance of certification. Achieving this recommendation will also require development of new strategies to measure important but difficult to assess competencies related to the following professional commitments:

   - To support the well-being of patients and populations;

   - To partner with patients and with colleagues from other professions to optimize health and health care;

- To remain ethical and professional in work habits and relationships, and

- To engage in continuous learning throughout one's career using reliable external assessments of personal performance to inform learning plans and continuing education.

3. Health care institutions that sponsor health professions education should track outcomes relevant to a high-performing health care system to ensure that the competency-based, time-variable educational programs are addressing critical societal needs. Specific outcomes that should be measured include the following:

   - Patient outcomes that can be correlated with a health professional's educational preparation (known as educationally sensitive patient outcomes), such as health literacy and active participation in care;

   - Health system outcomes related to the Quadruple Aim, including quality-of-care standards, patient experience measurements, population health costs of care, and measures of health professional well-being; and

   - Health professions workforce outcomes such as diversity and inclusivity of the health professions workforce and distribution of health professionals to optimize access to all people.

4. Accreditors of health professions educational institutions and organizations should develop organizational standards that support effective competency-based education. Critical standards should focus on the following:

   - Ensuring the adequacy of resources to support faculty development and faculty time spent in assessment and learning responsibilities.

- Demonstrating that faculty success is assessed using promotion and tenure processes that equally value and recognize excellence and impact in education, research, and clinical care.

5. Public and private partnerships should chart the course of and fund a national research agenda on competency-based, time-variable health professions education. Quantitative and qualitative methods should be used to conduct research in two general areas: 1) process studies at both individual and program levels; and 2) defining outcomes that are both proximal and distal to the learning experiences. Examples of areas in need of further study include the following:

- The entrustment decision-making process and the impact of entrustment on learning and care at the individual and program levels;

- Barriers to the implementation of competency-based, time-variable education, including issues related to feasibility, fidelity, and acceptability;

- Economic issues relevant to the conduct of competency-based educational programs; and

- Relationships between program inputs (such as human resources and technology), processes (such as organizational policies and curricula), and outcomes at individual and programmatic levels (individual outcomes should include a comparison of learners in competency-based, time-variable programs vs. traditional educational programs).

CONCLUSION

Improving health and health care will take more than redesigning the health care delivery system. It also requires changing the way those who work in that system are educated and trained. The Macy conferees strongly believe that this will require adopting a competency-based, time-variable educational model for health professionals across the continuum of their careers. In this model—which benefits learners, educators, practitioners, and patients—time becomes a resource rather than a restriction. Implementing such a model will take leadership at all levels, the development of a robust program of assessment, a commitment to research and innovation, a shifting of culture toward co-producing education, and resources devoted to education and educational research. In the end, we believe health professionals will be better prepared to meet patients' needs and more satisfied in their chosen careers. Health care will be more efficient and of higher quality, and society will be healthier.

The conclusions and recommendations from a Macy conference represent a consensus of the group and do not imply unanimity on every point. All conference members participated in the process, reviewed the final product, and provided input before publication. Participants are invited for their individual perspectives and broad experience and not to represent the views of any organization.

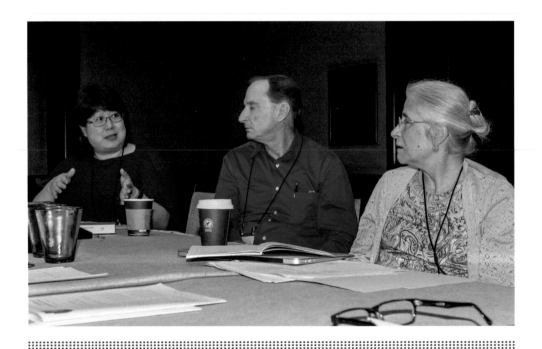

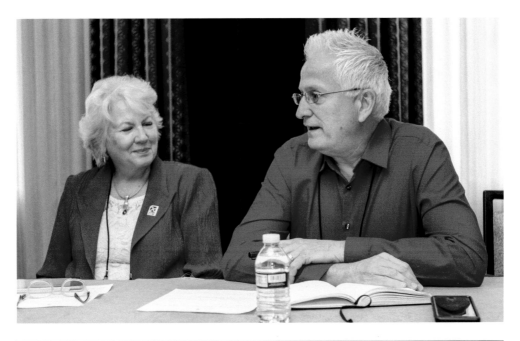

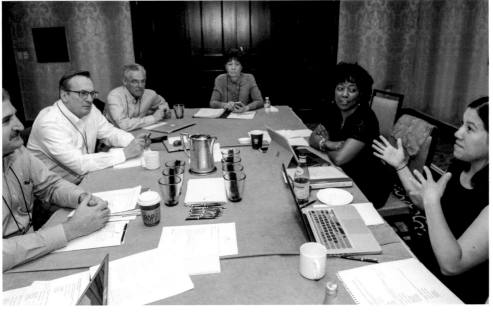

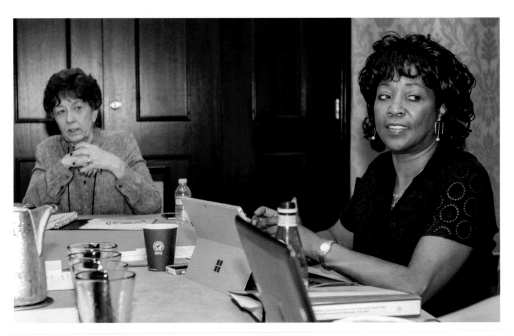

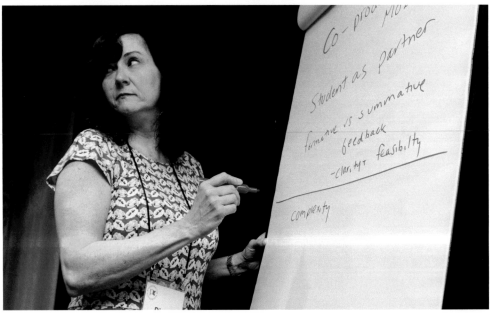

TIME-VARIABLE TRAINING IN MEDICINE:

INSIGHTS DERIVED FROM THE LITERATURE AND FROM EXAMPLES IN PRACTICE

Commissioned Paper

Olle ten Cate, PhD
Professor of Medical Education
Director, Center for Research and Development of Education
University Medical Center Utrecht, the Netherlands

Eugène J.F.M. Custers, PhD
Center for Research and Development of Education
University Medical Center Utrecht, the Netherlands

Larry D. Gruppen, PhD
Professor of Medical Education
Director of the Master of Health Professions Education Program
Department of Learning Health Sciences
University of Michigan Medical School

Lorelei Lingard, PhD
Founding Director & Senior Scientist, Center for Education Research & Innovation
Schulich School of Medicine and Dentistry, Western University, Ontario, Canada

Pim W. Teunissen, MD, PhD
Associate Professor
Maastricht University, the Netherlands

Jennifer R. Kogan, MD
Professor of Medicine
University of Pennsylvania Perelman School of Medicine

TABLE OF CONTENTS

Summary

1. Introduction

2. Theoretical and conceptual considerations for time-variable medical training

3. Context-dependence and time variability of clinical training

4. Time-variable medical training and the medical education continuum

5. The need for comprehensive learner assessment in time-variable medical training

5.1   The need for precision in assessment

5.2   The need for more continuous assessment

5.3   Context specificity of assessment

6. Legislative, regulatory and other system factors affecting training duration

6.1   Time-variable training and clinical service provision

6.2   Time-variable training, accreditation, and licensure

6.3   Time-variable training, credits, and tuition

7. Managing expectations related to time variability in training

7.1   Individual expectations

7.2   Institutional expectations

7.3   Societal expectations

8. Coda

SUMMARY

Time-variable medical training (TVMT)—defined as *the arrangement of an educational program to be variable in duration, at least in part depending on the progress a trainee makes, to ensure adequate competence at an individual's completion of the program*—has recently caught the interest of the medical education community related to the wide introduction of competency-based medical education, particularly in postgraduate training. A shift from "fixed time, variable outcomes" to "fixed outcomes, variable time" has been defended as a desirable target for the future of medical training.

In addition to the desire to control the outcome of training to ensure graduate competence, other rationales for time variability include a wish to accommodate other ambitions of trainees, such as building a research career, building a family, and potentially reducing training time. Historically, a critical discussion about the time required time to graduate has not occurred until way in the 20th century. In fact, time variability has been a dominant model across most of history. However, investigations to convincingly justify specific training lengths do not appear to have been conducted. Based on the authors' knowledge of the literature and known examples from practice, the current document was compiled to discuss time variability from theoretical, conceptual, and contextual angles, with respect to content, assessment, and regulation of education and training.

From the 1960s on, educational theory, such as the Carroll model and mastery learning, has provided a more general rationale for time variability in education. Other concepts relevant for TVMT, such as deliberate practice, neuroscience, motivation theories, entrustable professional activities, and identity formation are discussed. All these concepts support, to a certain extent, the feasibility and justification of time-variable training to gain more control over the outcome of training.

Next, the clinical context in which learning occurs is highlighted. Contexts vary in their affordance for learning and consequently in the time it takes to acquire competence. Shaping contexts for learning may be approached with different purposes. *Acquisition* and *participation* metaphors are used to contrast approaches, illustrating the creation of efficient blocks of time to enforce predefined learning experiences for knowledge and skills acquisition versus the practice of participating in health care responsibilities and more tacitly developing into a professional. The latter approach may include deliberate 'dwell time' that cannot always explicitly be linked to knowledge and skill acquisition, but nevertheless seems necessary for development and maturation. A most important component of the context is the teams learners work within. Team compositions may not benefit from frequent transitions of their members. Time-variable training with a focus on efficiency and time reduction may also predispose to stress and burnout. Potentially detrimental, unintended consequences of focusing on increased efficiency of training time in TVMT are discussed.

While TVMT is often discussed within the context of rotations or single programs, it may also be viewed from the perspective of the medical education continuum. There have been calls to reduce the total length of medical training and to streamline content (is it necessary to teach everything to everyone?) and reduce costs, particularly as medical student debt in the US training model has reached (too) high levels. Notably, however, there is no documentation of over-training, but there is documentation of perceived gaps in training and experience at the beginning of residency, fellowship, and unsupervised practice. Issues to consider for TVMT across the continuum include trainees' self-perceptions about their readiness to transition, dealing with trainees who transition but are actually not well-prepared (as is documented in the literature for some specialties), required flexibility in training programs and in workforce coverage when trainees deviate from time planning schedules, and communication of learner competence ("learner handoffs") across compartments of the continuum.

TVMT requires not only individualized training pathways, but also individualized and more continuous assessment efforts, including an infrastructure of regular sharing of progress data within clinical competency or entrustment committees (e.g., supported by an e-portfolio). The system will have to grapple with subjectivity (or organized tacit expert opinions) and context specificity in assessment if entrustment decisions become more dominant in the practice of learner evaluation. Mobile technology may be used for the collection of data in the natural course of clinical activities and the divide between formative and summative assessment may blur. This may be justified, but may not always be well-received by learners; documentation of suboptimal performance and its related feedback is a sensitive issue.

Moving to more TVMT will challenge regulations not only for service provision, but also for matching graduates into residency programs; allocation of credit hours, tuition, and related student debts; and accreditation and licensure. However, some small-scale projects (three-year undergraduate medical education programs; a pediatric continuum project) and existing training models in some countries show that attending to these is not impossible.

Finally, not unimportant in TVMT is the management of expectations among learners, clinical educators and program directors, institutions, and society. If "faster" becomes the norm, the primary purpose of TVMT is not realized. It is suggested that variations in time based on individual competence differences that exceed 20% (plus or minus) may not be considered adequate anymore. Finally, "longer" is not necessarily a sign of inadequate progression as time will also increase experience at the benefit of health care provision.

TVMT is an interesting and challenging topic, conceptually defendable, probably executable to a certain extent, but it requires a shift in thinking about medical education and definitely a shift in practice on various levels. Research will remain important, but finding conclusive evidence to guide decisions in medical education policy will be difficult, if possible at all.

1. INTRODUCTION

1.1 Origin and definition of time-variable medical training

Time-variable medical training has been a dominant issue in the discourse of medical education since about 2010, when the definition of competency-based medical education was explicitly proposed to stress standardization of outcomes to all trainees, de-emphasizing time-based training.[1,2] The idea of time-variable training was, however, not new. As Jason said back in 1969, "By making time a constant, we make achievement a variable. The most mature educational programs [..] specify objectives sufficiently clearly so that achievement can be made a constant, which in turn requires that time be made a variable."[3] In 1978, McGaghie et al. added some empirical underpinning, stating that "the principles of learning for mastery—i.e., entry-level testing, stepwise instruction, flexible time scheduling, and frequent assessment—describe the operational characteristics of the competency-based curriculum model [..]. When a combination of clinical problems, independent study, audiovisual materials, and computer-based mastery testing was used, Sorlie and co-workers reported that one group of medical students was able to satisfy basic sciences requirements, usually achieved after two years, in only one year."[4] This clearly refers to time variability among individual learners and increased efficiency of new instructional methods, albeit with respect to the basic sciences. Decades later, Long (2000), Carraccio (2002), and others alluded to this move from fixed-time-and-variable-outcomes to fixed-outcomes-and-variable-time.[4–6]

Time variability is but one aspect of competency-based medical education,[7,8] but it is the sole focus of this document. Time variability in medical training raises many questions. Schools, educators in undergraduate and postgraduate medical programs, and regulatory bodies seem to acknowledge its rationale and are interested in understanding it conceptually, but at the same time remain confused about the implications of applying the idea in practice. While the question *"How can we organize training to advance, graduate, or license a trainee at the moment the individual is ready for it?"* may not easily yield an unequivocal answer, a critical analysis is worth sharing. Time-variable medical training is a multifaceted issue that should be considered from a variety of angles.

This paper was commissioned to prepare for an expert meeting discussing time-variable training and "to provide examples how we can accomplish this in health professions education, [..] to identify challenges in moving to this approach, [to provide] suggestions for overcoming those challenges, [..] and to identify key areas that would benefit from recommendations." The aim of the project is to cover a broad range of aspects and arguments in order to enable a rich discussion and policy development in medical education at local, national, and international levels.

For the purpose of this paper, we will use the acronym TVMT (time-variable medical training) and apply the following definition: time-variable training is *the arrangement of an educational program to be variable in duration, at least in part depending on the progress a trainee makes, to ensure adequate competence at an individual's completion of the program.* Variation also may apply to the number of hours of education within a given duration, in case of a less than full-time program. Limits to this variation may be set in terms of minimum and maximum durations. Reasons for variation may be pre-existing knowledge and skills, individual capabilities and learning opportunities during the training period, foreseen or unforeseen interruptions in the program, and other conditions. We consider time variation to pertain essentially to clinical (i.e., individual) workplace curricula, but time variation in classroom courses will be discussed too.

1.2 Historical notes

While accounts from ancient history show the existence of medical training, formal medical education started in Europe in the Middle Ages. From approximately 1100 to 1800, the medical profession was practiced in Europe by two types of professionals: the university-educated *Doctores Medicinae* and the apprenticeship-trained (*barber-*) *surgeons*. Universities had little to no performance criteria for graduation, and education could be completed in as little two years after a preparatory education that would also take two years. Surgeons could be trained within highly esteemed guilds, which included anatomical lessons, botany, and extensive supervised training in practice up to five years, such as in the Amsterdam Guild of Surgeons, and concluded with a "master piece" examination. Guilds were predominantly economical units, apprentices were workforce, and training varied greatly among different guilds.[*]

After the French Revolution, medical education changed as guilds were gradually abandoned and university education evolved into curricula with required courses. The Netherlands established "clinical schools" that existed for a few decades. Only in the second half of the 19th century did national legislations begin to require both university education and practical training to allow the privilege of patient care. While the content of medical education became defined in European schools, its length was often not critical, and left to however long it took learners to complete the requirements, often with infinite opportunities to retake exams. Anecdotal descriptions from Dutch education show vast variations in training length and far from optimal completion rates until well after World War II, in contrast with US medical education with its fixed classes and duration.

US medical education has a shorter history and was not organized in guilds. An extended preceptorship was the dominant model of medical education until the mid-19th century, and medical schools, most weakly organized, offered programs of two or three years, reflecting differences in both admission criteria and outcomes. While clinical training was part of many programs, it was not necessary until the early 20th century. In 1919 the American Medical Association demanded internships; however, internships could vary in length from 12 to 36 months. After WWII, four-year medical schools had become standard, with clerkships to obtain clinical experience, but since the 1950s complaints that four years were inadequate could

---

[*] Based on a manuscript that is being prepared in conjunction with the current document: Custers EJFM, ten Cate O. Historical aspects of medical education with respect to time and proficiency in Europe and North America.

be heard, and many students chose rotating internships after medical school to widen their experience. From the 1950s onward, the increasing overload of content in medical schools was becoming a burden that required schools to integrate and rethink the time needed to prepare for residency. Early proposals for time-variable training emerged from the 1970s on.[3,4]

Meanwhile, postgraduate medical training, first established at John Hopkins University by William Osler and William Halsted,[9] became a requirement for most practitioners and a benchmark to define the length of undergraduate training. In 1975, the European Economic Community (EEC) determined that a prerequisite for any speciality training in EEC countries was the completion of a six-year undergraduate program or 5,500 hours of theoretical and practical training, including "suitable clinical experience in hospitals."[10] This requirement was continued until 2013, when six years was decreased to "at least five years" of undergraduate training.[11] The same EEC directive has also defined medical specialties with their minimum training lengths to enable an open European Union labor market. The directive probits the assessment of international graduates from other EU countries, in an attempt to avoid any obstacles in the EU labor market. Programs have often created specialty programs that exceed these minimum lengths.

History has not given a clear rationale for the need of any specific length of training for medicine or for a given specialty. The length of training is basically an arbitrary and historically and politically agreed upon entity that proved workable, but that never had an empirically argued grounding. As to the strictness of program lengths in Europe, in the past century, the European tendency has been towards greater leniency and flexibility than North America.

1.3   General rationales for time-variable medical training

The most important rationale for TVMT and outcome-based curricula has been to define standards for graduation that are more or less fixed, to ensure quality and safety of medical practice. Given a presumed variation among trainees, because of ability, circumstances, or both, it is considered unlikely that all trainees meet these standards at the same time. As a result, an important rationale for time variability in training is a better control of competence at graduation while simultaneously catering to the needs of individual learners.[2] This includes a quality issue to protect the public against unsafe practice.

A second rationale for a competency-based postgraduate medical education system based on variable time is increasing educational efficiency at the individual level. Several authors have voiced the desire to decrease the total length of medical training.[12,13] While the assumption that TVMT *may* reduce training time must be investigated and is conceptually not the purpose of time variability, some examples show such reduction in time may happen across cohorts of learners. However, program time reduction may occur at the cost of a higher intensity of supervision.[14–17] In other words, the increased educational efficiency at an individual level (i.e., an individual learner may finish early) may have to be paid for at a system level, by more faculty investment in supervision and organizational disutility due to health care planning issues because one cannot assume residents will be on the roster for a fixed time. A focus on time *reduction* may also inadvertently corrupt outcome-based curricula's aim to ensure high-quality training results when it leads to working toward a minimally acceptable level. Having said that, regulatory and funding bodies may pursue policies that link competency-based education to a general reduction in time.

> **Box 1.1 Time variability induced by national policy: a Dutch example**
>
> A recent cut on government funding for Dutch postgraduate medical programs has led all programs to seek flexibility and individualization, assuming that *on average*, the length of training will decrease and consequently training costs. This policy has led to more or less forced deliberations about TVMT within the community. In 2014, the Dutch College of Medical Specialties adapted regulations of postgraduate medical training to allow for 'individualisation of training length" (https://vimeo.com/178895320) as a result of this government policy.

A third rationale for TVMT is the wish to accommodate activities other than medical training within the training period. This wish tends to lead to a hybrid model where the total volume of training time remains fixed. Depending on an individual learner's progression, additional time is allocated for personal development that goes beyond standard curricular outcomes, such as research, or even to non-work related demands, such as family building, which can lead to additional training time. For example, research during medical training has become increasingly commonplace. Combined MD-PhD or residency-PhD programs have been created to foster the education of clinician scientists, but combining the two training objectives (medicine and science) has not been easy. Individually tailored programs have been recommended.[18,19] Additionally, the percentage of female residents having children during training has reportedly tripled in the past three decades, and 40% of residents now plan to raise a family during residency.[20] At the same time, the ratio of females to males in training has increased.[21] Work-life balance has become an important concern among medical trainees. It not only affects career choice,[22] but an adequate balance is also felt to decrease the risk of burn-out and depression among medical students and residents.[23,24] Time-variable training arrangements may serve to create a feasible work-life balance.

1.4   Methods of investigation

The authors considered conducting a systematic review, as was initially commissioned, but this approach seemed inadequate to capture the richness of, and variations in, reasons and implications of TVMT. Furthermore, given that TVMT initiatives may be nascent, existing examples from practice may be relevant, even if they are not well documented in the scientific literature. Therefore, the approach to this project was to select experienced medical educators as a writing team, generate as many relevant facets of TVMT as possible, and ground general insights and conclusions in the literature and case examples.

One author with expertise in the history of medical education (EC) was asked to provide a historical overview of time variability and its rationale in medical education in Europe and North America to serve as a separate background document. The other authors were first asked to generate initial thoughts to enable an overview for an outline of the document. This first led to an unstructured seven-page document from which the first author extracted themes that were shared with all other authors, with the request to add to or amend the list.

Next, themes were redistributed among the authors; each author took primary ownership of one or more themes in collaboration with one or two other authors. Authors searched for literature and examples from practice and drafted paragraphs for the current document. The full document was edited (by OtC) and shared among the authors for approval and extension, if necessary.

A first analysis of the topic by the authoring team led to the identification of various themes. Some were combined; others were elaborated in sub-sections and redistributed over the paper to establish coherence and minimize duplication of arguments. A full draft was shared which led to significant comments and reorganization of the paper.

2. THEORETICAL AND CONCEPTUAL CONSIDERATIONS FOR TVMT

Billett reminds us how training in the professions in the pre-school era of history all happened in the workplace[25] and likely in a time-variable, individualized fashion. Modern societies have regulated the content and length of medical training programs. Yet the rationale underpinning the length chosen has never been well argued from a theoretical point of view. This section cannot provide this rationale, but attempts to discuss theoretical and conceptual aspects that relate to time needed for training, with particular reference to variability tailored to the individual learner. Educational theory, particularly from the 1960s on, has provided general rationales to such variability in education through the Carroll model and mastery learning. Other concepts relevant for TVMT, such as deliberate practice, neuroscience, motivation theories, entrustable professional activities, and identity formation, are discussed.

2.1 *Time* in the equation of educational theory – the Carroll model

The roots of competency- and outcomes-based education, conceptually linked to time variability, may be found in the early post-war educational thinking that emerged around educational objectives, initiated by Ralph Tyler[26] and followed by Benjamin Bloom's work elaborating taxonomies of objectives for education.[27,28] Tyler proposed that schools should rethink their purpose and organize experiences of learners toward those purposes.[29] He worked intimately with Case Western Reserve University to define objectives for medical training. Once objectives for education became accepted, John B. Carroll, an educational psychologist, proposed a model that included aptitude, perseverance, and quality of instruction, saying that the "degree of learning = f(Time Spent/Time Needed), or, in other words, "the learner will succeed in learning a given task to the extent that he spends the amount of time that he needs to learn the task."[30,31] This general thinking has been applied to medical training in an early stage.[3]

2.2 Time variability from the perspective of mastery learning, deliberate practice, and learning curves

The Carroll model inspired Bloom to develop a model of education called "mastery learning,"[32] a concept that quickly caught the attention of medical educators.[4] Mastery learning outcomes are meant to be uniform with little or no variation among learners. By contrast, educational time can vary among learners. McGaghie explains seven conditions for mastery learning:[33]

- Baseline or entry-level diagnostic testing

- Clear learning objectives, sequenced as units usually in increasing difficulty

- Engagement in educational activities (e.g., deliberate skills practice, calculations, data interpretation, reading) focused on reaching the objectives

- A set minimum passing standard (e.g., test score) for each educational unit

- Formative testing to gauge unit completion at a preset minimum passing standard for mastery

- Advancement to the next educational unit given measured achievement at or above the mastery standard

- Continued practice or study on an educational unit until the mastery standard is reached.

The time variation as a necessary component of mastery learning is captured in the seventh feature ". . . until the mastery standard is reached," which supposedly will be different for various learners.

Mastery learning is rooted in behaviorist principles and established most of its success in the 1980s. In fact, it is one of the most studied educational methods and its learning effects are well documented, particularly in the cognitive domain.[34,35] With the expansion of simulation techniques, mastery learning has enjoyed a revival in medical education.[36–38]

Mastery learning has close similarity with deliberate practice, an educational principle developed and studied by Ericsson, defined as engagement in structured activities created specifically to improve performance in a domain.

Compared with mastery learning, which is cognitively oriented, deliberate practice is usually focused on skills (sports, chess, musical proficiency, surgical or procedural skill) and includes several conditions that must be met:[39]

- Motivated learners with good concentration

- Well-defined learning objectives or tasks with appropriate level of difficulty

- Focused, repetitive practice

- Rigorous, reliable measurements of results

- Informative feedback (e.g., from simulators or teachers)

- Monitoring, error correction, and subsequent further practice

- Mastery standards where learning time may vary, but expected minimal outcomes are identical

- Advancement to the next task or unit with higher standards if previous standards are met.

In a recent meta-analysis, it was concluded that the deliberate practice approach is particularly successful in games, music, and sport, but hardly successful in education and in professions.[40] For medicine, this may be explained by the fact that, in the clinical workplace, the focus of effort of learners may be more on completing patient care tasks than on deliberate practice toward achieving learning goals.[41] Medicine is highly uncertain, constantly dynamic, and requires an adaptive expertise rather than "routine" expertise. Deliberate practice in most of medicine does not fit the idea of practicing an arpeggio on a musical instrument over and over until it is perfect. Each medical case or "arpeggio" is different from the next. Outside the workplace however, e.g. in simulation labs, deliberate practice has shown to be effective.[38,39]

In some areas of medicine, the relation between practice effort and proficiency has been well-established. One example is gaining competency in colonoscopy procedures. Figure 2.1 below, from Chung and colleagues,[42] shows typical learning curves of 12 fellows based on 3.243 colonoscopies. The authors concluded that at their center 200 colonoscopies are necessary to attain the proficiency to conduct them in a reasonable time, but individual differences can readily be seen.

Figure 2.1 Number of colonoscopies to attain proficiency

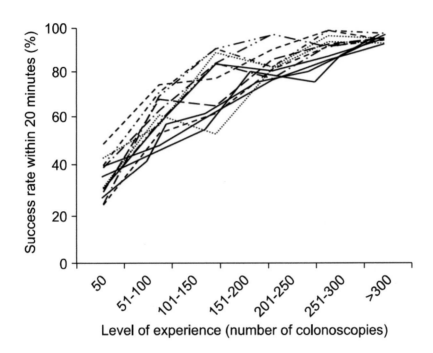

Open access publication, permission to reuse for non-commercial purposes

The conclusion is that competency-based education or time-variable training is not in conflict with setting minimum quality standards for training.[43] Pusic and colleagues have suggested that, in time-based curricula, the cut-off divide in such learning curves represents a vertical line, whereas in competency-based curricula this is a horizontal line (as will be discussed later in Figure 2.4).[44]

Figure 2.2 shows scores on a Dutch national formative radiology progress test that was administered biannually to all residents across five programs years, from April 2005 to April 2009.[45] The projected lines represent a recent discussion to transition to a summative examination with a cut-off score that all residents should meet.

Most residents will have passed this threshold after three years, but some fifth year residents currently do not meet that criterion at the end of training and require remediation (the shaded block), following a shift toward a competency-based program.

Figure 2.2 2006–2009 progress test scores of Dutch radiology residents PGY1 to PGY5

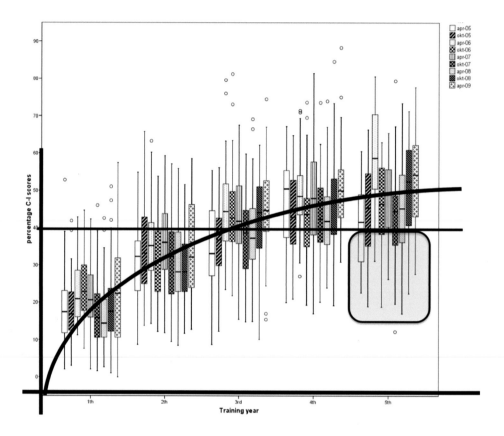

Cecile Ravesloot, Marieke van der Schaaf, Cees Haaring, et al. Construct validation of progress testing to measure knowledge and visual skills in radiology. Med Teach. 2012;34(12): 1044-1075. Reprinted by permission of Taylor & Francis Ltd, www.tandfonline.com

2.3 Neuroscience of time and learning

It has been well established in neuroscience that learning (i.e., the adaptation of the brain) does not only happen during deliberate learning activities. Brain development also happens in informal or implicit (i.e., not-planned) learning and in subsequent periods of rest. Sleep fosters memory consolidation.[46–49] It is also known that for learning goals requiring extensive practice, spaced practice over prolonged time is more effective than massed practice in a condensed time, despite similar investment of practice hours.[50–53] Evidently, something happens in periods of non-practice that contributes to a learning effect, akin to muscle development after physical training. Time-variable programs should therefore consider the importance of time needed that is not filled with learning activities, at least not with repetition of similar activities in a short period of time, and the importance of mental rest for learning. Anecdotal reports suggest that residents who have been permitted to work for four instead of five days per week to allow for child rearing seem not to lag behind in their development (R Hoff, director of anesthesiology residency program at UMC Utrecht, personal communication, 2017).

2.4 Time variability and theories of motivation

Agency of learners is dependent on their motivation to act. In clinical workplaces, self-regulation of learning is key in the development of competence, much more than in preclinical classroom teaching. Hence, individual variation in the time it takes to develop competence may in part be explained by motivation and self-regulated learning ability. While motivation may in part be a characteristic of an individual, motivation is also affected by contextual factors and emotions that in turn affect achievement.[54,55] Therefore, a discussion of motivation theories is warranted; we briefly focus on goal orientation and self-determination theories.

Goal orientation theory

From the literature it is clear how valuable a learning goal orientation is for learning from challenging situations. Someone with a goal of learning (a *mastery goal orientation*) is less focused on performance and is more concerned with gaining new knowledge and skills. On the other hand, someone with a goal of performance (a *performance goal orientation*) is focused on winning positive and avoiding negative judgments of one's competence.[56] Outcome-based curricula that focus on attaining a required level of performance carry the risk of preferentially strengthening a performance goal orientation in learners, particularly in medicine's competitive learning culture, with the possibility that additional time in the same context after reaching (minimum) standards could be considered wasted time or a sign of less capability in a competitive world.[57]

As discussed in a later section, however, a trainee's context almost always has the potential to offer new challenges or other learning opportunities. Trainees can be helped, even taught, to continuously set achievement goals in line with their ambitions, even when tasks feel routine, so as to promote additional professional development.[58] Having to learn from routine work and not fall prey to the risk of becoming an *experienced non-expert* resembles actual practice and therefore helps prepare learners for post-training continuing professional development. A good time for a learner to move on may be when the learner, supervisor, and other co-workers feel that there remains little to gain in learning anymore. One important caveat in reasoning is that learning may be implicit and invisible, but still adds to important experience.

Self-determination theory

Self-determination theory (SDT) is another major motivational theory. SDT is explained in a series of principles, one of which is the distinction of three innate psychological needs of human beings that must be satisfied to generate and maintain intrinsic motivation: a feeling of competence, a feeling of autonomy, and a feeling of relatedness to a group or community, such as friends, family, or colleagues.

A clinical context that satisfies these needs—by rewarding competence, granting responsibilities when possible, providing autonomy at work (i.e., by accepting learners as important members of the health care team)—can be expected to foster intrinsic motivation, achievement, and well-being.[59] Self determination and intrinsic motivation may lead to more individualized learning paths requiring variations between learners.

2.5 Time variability and entrustable professional activities

The concept of entrustable professional activities (EPAs; units of professional practice to be entrusted to learners for unsupervised execution once they have demonstrated sufficient competence) was created to link competencies to everyday practice and implies time variability. As not all EPAs are mastered at the level of unsupervised practice at the end of training (or, for undergraduate medical education, at the level of indirect supervision), the reasoning is that EPAs foster the deliberate granting of responsibilities as soon as learners are ready for them. As training progresses, trainees may thus become gradually qualified and entitled to perform EPAs and transform from a trainee into a professional.[60] To account for individual differences in the time to master EPAs, individualized training pathways and time variability may be necessary.[61] This time variability is not necessarily meant to decrease or increase the total length of training, but rather to ensure learners only start working on tasks unsupervised when they can handle them. If across all essential EPAs of a program this means that the confidence in learners is established early, a decrease in total length may be possible, but it is just as reasonable to expect that some learners will require an increase in total time.

However, one of the key aspects of EPA-based workplace curricula is that learners experience working with full responsibility and autonomy while still in training, with only distant supervision, before they graduate to independent practice. If a learner graduates a program having received close supervision until the last day of training, that student may feel too insecure and unprepared to start working unsupervised.[62,63] Figure 2.3 shows what, for a given trainee, a portfolio of EPAs may look like.[64] EPA a is expected to be mastered at the "indirect supervision" (Level 3) in the first half of postgraduate Year 3. Expectations are that this learner will be ready for unsupervised practice (Level 4) in the second half, and able to supervise this EPA (Level 5) a year later. Careful monitoring of this trainee may lead to adaptation of the initially planned moments of entrustment.

Figure 2.3 A schematic part-portfolio of EPAs at various supervision levels

Portfolio of : Trainee Jones	PGY1		PGY2		PGY3		PGY4	
EPA a	1	2	2	2	3	4	4	5
EPA b	1	1	2	2	2	3	3	4
EPA c	2	2	3	4	5	5	5	5
EPA d	2	3	4	4	4	4	5	5

Reproduced from a chart originally appearing in Academic Medicine Last Page.

Wiersma et al. recently reported how portfolios of 101 physician assistants (PAs) in training appeared highly indivdualized and flexible using EPAs.[65] In this program, each PA student has a unique set of EPAs to be mastered. Trainees had, on average, curricula with about 7 EPAs, of which 1.5 changed across 2.5 years of training, based on their experience and need for training within the context of the clinical department in which they were placed. If a trainee masters *all* core EPAs of a program sooner (or later), then an adaptation of the overall length of training seems indicated.

However, there is another route to the desired variation. Variability can also be created through the combined core *and* variable elective EPAs the learner is to master by the end of training. When considering EPAs and TVMT, the variables are not only time and competence, but also the breadth of the portfolio of EPAs of a trainee. Trainees may all graduate at an adequate (minimum) level of competence, but with more or fewer elective EPAs added to their portfolio. When moving to next stages of a career, EPAs may be added or may be lost after periods of non-practice, which could make this portfolio a dynamic reflection of actual competence in practice.[66]

Figure 2.4 schematically depicts how, for a given EPA, somewhere along a developmental trajectory the learner appears ready for unsupervised practice. A summative entrustment decision as an informal certification, which may be preceded by a supervisor's making multiple satisfactory *ad hoc* entrustment decisions situationally, is not necessarily made at the end of the training period. In other words, for different EPAs, different moments in time may allow for a justified summative entrustment decision for unsupervised practice. From that moment on, distant supervision or clinical oversight may suffice until the end of training (the rimmed box). The shadings indicate decreasing supervision as training progresses: (1) the learner observing only, (2) the learner enacting the EPA with direct supervision in the room, (3) with indirect supervision not in the room but quickly available, (4) with distant supervision not quickly available. While using this training model may require adequate levels of permission for actual care delivery, the message is that a gradual growth of responsibility, rather than an abrupt transition at the moment of licensing, may enhance the process of becoming a legitimate member of a professional community.

Figure 2.4 Graduated levels of supervision on a developmental trajectory for an EPA

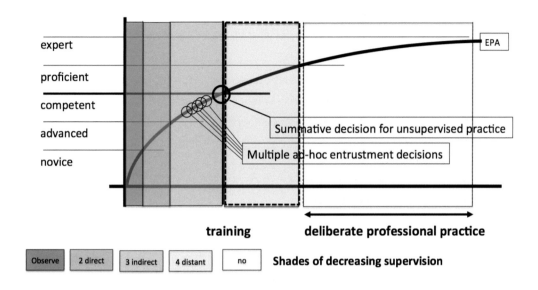

While the concept of EPAs was originally created to operationalize competency-based education in postgraduate training and, in that context, to enable more variability in the trajectory to unsupervised practice, undergraduate medical education is beginning to embrace the concept too.[67,68] In addition, EPAs have recently been suggested to be a suitable vehicle to bridge the divides between undergraduate and graduate medical education (UME, GME) and perhaps also continuing medical education (CME).[69] While these are speculations at the moment, EPAs may facilitate time variability across the continuum in the future.

2.6 Time variability from the perspective of identity formation

Professional identity of the physician has been defined as "a representation of self, achieved in stages over time during which the characteristics, values, and norms of the medical profession are internalized, resulting in an individual *thinking, acting, and feeling like a physician.*"[70] Time-variable training from the perspective of knowledge and skill, as exemplified in mastery learning, does not take into account that professional development may take time, independent of skill development. As Hafferty noted, "while any occupational training involves learning new knowledge and skills, it is the melding of knowledge and skills with an altered sense of self that differentiates socialization from training."[71] Individuals differ in the time this process of identity formation takes, and educational programs can affect that process, but the dynamics may be quite different from the acquisition of knowledge and skills.[72] For instance, rituals in medical training, such as white coat ceremonies and the actual awarding of a medical degree, and the granting of responsibilities in patient care, such as with deliberate entrustment decisions,[73] are likely to influence a learner's sense of socialization into the profession.

This may even be an ongoing process as physicians assume broader responsibilities. Any training program that has a specified end (time-fixed or time-variable) will graduate learners who will continue to develop in their identity. Identity formation is not easily captured in any specific time framing, but may be hampered when substantial shortening of training occurs and learners must act as professionals while not feeling ready for it. It is an area for future research as to how identity formation (1) is affected by time variation and (2) relates to quality of care.

3. CONTEXT-DEPENDENCE AND TIME VARIABILITY OF CLINICAL TRAINING

In a time when virtually all health care was learned in practice settings, Plato wrote, "the best physicians are those who have treated the greatest number of constitutions good and bad."[25] Extensive clinical experience with many different patients with variable clinical problems seems conditional for the acquisition of clinical expertise. Medical competence requires training in a clinical context, and contexts may vary in how they afford opportunities to learn.[74] This accords with the fact that clinical reasoning ability draws heavily on the recognition of patterns and a repository of illness scripts represented in long-term memory built over time.[75,76] Before answering the question of how learning in practice can benefit from time variability, the relationship between context and learning should be examined.

3.1 The impact of the clinical context on learning

The clinical workplace typically combines a deliberate curricular intent with what has been called a "hidden" curriculum. The hidden curriculum refers to cultural mores that are transmitted, but not openly acknowledged, through formal and informal educational practices.[77] Hafferty and Hafler acknowledge that "workplace learning is truly extraordinary when it is marked by a structural congruence [..] between the intended and formal preparation of professionals, the tacit learning [..] in the hidden curriculum, and the [..] demands embedded in subsequent workplace setting."[78] They conclude, however, that congruence between curricular intentions and practice in the clinical enviroment seldom align and recommend better shaping clinical environments for learning. Some clinical workplaces may simply yield better learning effects than others.[79,80] This raises the question of whether curricular organization could enable this alignment.

Contexts are often assigned up front (i.e., the beginning of an academic year) and are not iteratively adjusted based on learners' needs. In theory, trainees could strategically be put in contexts that both support and challenge particular competencies. Next, contexts could be conceptualized not only as having clinical foci (e.g., core pediatrics, critical care), but also as having learning affordances reflective of different workplace dynamics, for instance, by creating relational continuity or fluidity among team members (e.g., the stable team membership of a pediatric burns unit versus the fluid team membership of an internal medicine ward). In practical terms, team members could be co-located or distributed (e.g., the shared physical space of the critical care unit versus the referral from family medicine to surgery). Such features strongly shape what constitutes competent team performance, and trainees would arguably benefit from experiencing these variable contexts according to a conscious educational strategy rather than a random rotation assignment.[81] Furthermore, clinical contexts could be conceptualized as those with trainee-patient continuity versus fragmentation (e.g., a longitudinal outpatient continuity clinic versus an emergency setting).

Two sets of advanced competencies could be refined by strategically selecting contexts to support and challenge them. The first begins to approach what has been called "collective competence," or the degree to which learners can recognize their place in the larger system of a unit or team, and strategically adapt their behaviors according to features such as team stability and trust.[82] The second moves beyond the individual patient encounter to address how learners assess and adapt to patient encounters with varying degrees of system continuity or fragmentation. The opportunity to use contexts strategically to expose and support such competencies would move us closer to inculcating in learners an awareness of these differences in systems of care and supporting learners to apply and adapt their skills in communication and collaboration accordingly. The experience of participating in different kinds of team contexts should also be considered and strategically organized to advance learning: teams range from discipline-specific (e.g., medicine) to interdisciplinary (e.g., family health team), and from co-located (e.g., operating room) to distributed (e.g., palliative care).

Contexts could also be used variously as learners acquire particular competencies. If a surgical trainee has acquired the technical competencies associated with general surgery, they could turn more attention to relational competencies, such as negotiating post-operative management with other specialties or leading family meetings in challenging clinical situations. Often, learners struggle to attend to such relational dimensions of clinical practice until the biomedical and technical dimensions are mastered. Dwell time is important not only to consolidate knowledge and skills, but also to allow learners to "graduate" to relational and social aspects of their situated expertise.[83,84]

Time needed in clinical education may thus depend on the provision and availability of clinical experiences and how they are perceived. These experiences can be far from optimal. Indeed, clinical education, particularly in tertiary hospitals, arguably suffers, more than in the past, from fragmentation of disciplines; short patient stays; frequent handoffs; short rotations; and inadequate supervision, observation, and teaching—all of which make the learning process complex.[85,86] Park and colleagues conclude that a shift from time-based to competency-based education is recommended, but is not easily achievable, predominantly because of the complexity of assessment in the workplace.[87] A short-cycled, rotational system of clinical education may hamper the ability to validly establish enough confidence in learners' competence to allow for time variability,[88–90] and restructuring clinical experiences into more longitudinal arrangements has been recommended.[91,92] Hirsh and others have recommended continuity as an organizing principle of clinical education,[89] moving from short rotations to longitudinal experiences to enable better guidance, assessment, and the building of preceptor-trainee trust relationships, in turn fostering better assessment possibilities for progression of learners.[88,93,94]

Adaptive expertise, performance, or competence has been stressed as an important 21st century skill for graduates,[95–97] to enable coping with a variety of contexts and unfamiliar situations. Training to acquire this would require experience in a variety of clinical settings. Together with the suggestion to move away from short rotations to more longitudinal clinical experiences as elaborated in the previous section, this would advocate longer rather than shorter training. Research is needed to establish when repetition of experiences adds productively to the development of competence and when it becomes redundant.

3.2 Learning as participating in the clinical workplace

Before considering TVMT in an outcome-based educational model, it is necessary to have a better understanding of the intimate relationship between learner, context, and competence.[98] It will be important to conceptualize a TVMT paradigm in which context is purposefully considered as a lever to advance competence. As such, what would it mean to conceptualize TVMT not exclusively as an individual timeline, but more broadly as a situated process in which context could be used to strategically develop and enhance learning? Crucial in the discussion about the possibilities and pitfalls of TVMT is one's epistemological orientation on how people learn in the clinical workplace. An *acquisition metaphor* of learning—focusing on individual, cognitive, and technical-rational aspects of learning—positions us to frame the discussion on TVMT as a matter of individuals attaining required objectives while the educational system adjusts to their differing pace of attainment.

This orientation, however, deflects attention from the role of context—the organizational system, clinical unit, or health care team. The acquisition metaphor of learning is problematic for learning in the clinical workplace. It tends to treat context as a temporal and spatial backdrop: clinical rotations, therefore, get conceptualized as blocks of time that trainees spend in particular places. This is exemplified by a fixed set of learning objectives for all trainees in a similar program (for instance, a medicine rotation in undergraduate medical education or an obstetrics/gynecology residency program in postgraduate medical education) regardless of the specific workplace setting. The pursuit to ensure that all learners attain fixed standards in competency-based medical education, with or without time variability for individuals, may increase pressure on learning contexts to become more uniform. Seeking uniformity of context not only could be dangerously artificial in a world of richly diverse clinical workplaces, but also could risk robbing clinical training of a powerful tool for advancing learner competence—the rich variability of workplace contexts.[99]

A great strength of workplace learning is that it offers learners unique access to the specific learning opportunities that a department, clinic, practice, etc., has to offer. However, this opportunity stands in contrast to a model of education that aims for standardization of outcomes for all trainees regardless of where they are trained. TVMT could be a tool that allows learners to flexibly use training time to benefit from the uniqueness of a workplace. On the other hand, TVMT could potentially result in increased uniformity of assessment and learning outcomes and devalue workplaces as learning environments.

In contrast, the *participation metaphor* of learning, which understands learning as situated, relational, and participatory, views context as having an integral influence on learning.[100] Adding this participatory orientation to discussions of TVMT allows for critical and strategic engagement of the influence of context in clinical training. After the early classroom years, medical training takes place in the clinical workplace through apprenticeship as part of a health care team delivering patient care. Theories of participatory learning have been used to understand and shape medical training. Each workplace context offers unique learning opportunities, and research shows that learners learn what a workplace has to offer through the experience of participating in patient care, regardless of what is included in the actual written curriculum.[101]

Competence emerges in the relationship between the learner and the situated exigencies of the work, including patient presentations, collaborative interactions, and organizational structures and policies. Thus there is a need for training programs that capitalize on contextual variation and expect and support learners to become sensitive to their practice context and to develop the context-bound competence required of them. The ability to adapt and refine competence to context is a critical dimension of lifelong learning, and it cannot be learned if contexts are treated as backdrops, preferably uniform, for the efficient acquisition of generic, minimum standards. Time-variable programs may adapt to such context variations better than programs with fixed time.[96,102]

Generally, these conceptualizations of workplace learning go beyond the boundaries of an individual's cognition.[103] They recognize the importance of the social nature of meaning making, the contextual influences on learners' developmental trajectories, and the plethora of cultural affordances in which learners are embedded.[99,104]

3.3 The significance of "dwell time"

Meeting minimum standards set by an outcomes- or competency-based curriculum does not equate to having exhausted the learning potential of the work context, nor does it necessarily imply a trainee is well-prepared for the next phase of training.[105] While outcomes-based education has the potential to offer clear learning goals for trainees, it is questionable whether everything that matters in a trainees' development can be captured in clear learning goals. Arguably, even the most granular set of objectives will not be able to capture the whole development from novice medical student to competent physician.[106,107] Therefore, TVMT may permit learners who have met minimum objectives to use additional time in a clinical context for refinement and maturation of more sophisticated and nuanced capabilities.

The direction of further development will vary between different learner-context combinations. It is important, though, that there is additional time to learn in the context where a trainee has reached the required level of competence and maturity necessary for relatively independent practice. This time has been called "dwell time"[93,108,109] or "tea steeping,"[110] as if a learner's development is idle in this period or happens unguided. On the contrary, we would characterize dwelling as guided transition to independence that can add significantly to developing well-rounded, adaptable professionals. It may be deliberately organized as reflective periods strategically inserted into a curriculum to foster deeper thinking and integration of knowledge, techniques, and their application to experiential learning.

Crucially, part of what develops through dwell time are social relationships. And as the relationship develops between a learner who has gradually moved from a peripheral participant to a full participant in the community of practice, new learning opportunities emerge.[104] The first opportunity relates to confidence and self-efficacy. Meeting standards may not always translate into learner confidence. But if a trusting relationship has developed,[93] supervisors may allow the learner to practice with guided independence, which presents the learner an opportunity to develop a sense of self-efficacy. This period—the rimmed box in figure 2.4—may not be specifically focused on gaining new competencies, but on consolidating existing performance.

The second learning opportunity has to do with the experience of failure. It is in the initial period after being entrusted with a professional activity that a fragile sense of certainty may be shattered by a mistake or a negative patient outcome. With an increase in one's volume of independent practice, it is inevitable that there will be times where a junior consultant has to take responsibility for something that didn't go as planned. This may be something seemingly minor, such as a laboratory test that wasn't ordered or a diagnostic error leading to prolonged suffering. Or it may be a major calamity, such as a surgical complication resulting in a patient's death.

It makes good educational sense to let trainees experience some of these initial moments of struggle in a context where they have the established relationships in place for both guided independence and mentored reflection.[111]

In such a context, trainees would have the social support of known colleagues, the advice of a supervisor who can act as a mentor or coach, and the certainty that they had acquired the trust needed to be the caregiver for the patient and the maturity to take responsibility for the unexpected outcome. How we teach young doctors to cope with the emotional, organizational, and potentially legal ramifications of situations that go awry will impact the rest of their careers. Helping physicians deal with challenges constructively and develop strategies for resiliency is possible only when there is the time and trust in place for the guided independence that produces such learning opportunities.

3.4 Potential effects of time variability on team work and well-being

Team collaboration

A TVMT model that urges learners to progress as soon as targets have been met may have negative consequences. Time in context after having reached a minimum required level of entrustment not only serves the individual, but also impacts the composition of the team at work in a clinical learning environment. Medical training is characterized by significant peer and near peer education. TVMT could reduce the number of competent learners available for (near) peer teaching that might otherwise occur during dwell time. Teams, as a whole, would generally have more novice members. Therefore, TVMT (particularly early completion of training) influences not only an individual learner, but also the learning environment of the team by removing competent learners who would have historically contributed to teaching more novice team members.

Burn-out and depression

The prevalence of burn-out and depression among medical trainees is higher than in comparable populations and appears to be increasing.[23,24,112] While general societal factors likely contribute to this (e.g., an increased need for competition and a strong desire to combine work with other goals in life), the clinical context may also contribute. Increased control and regulatory requirements in health care, tighter work hour regulations, and decreased autonomy of learners over the past decades[62,113] may contribute to a context in which learners feel more stressed. Time-variable training may lead to aggravation of these effects if learners were to feel the need to progress as fast as possible—i.e., if a decrease in training time were valued over an increase in training time.

4. TIME-VARIABLE MEDICAL TRAINING FROM THE PERSPECTIVE OF THE MEDICAL EDUCATION CONTINUUM

4.1 Efforts to reduce the length of the medical education continuum

During the past century, average time spent in training has considerably increased as unsupervised practice is hardly possible anymore without a specialty registration. In Western countries, the significance of attaining a medical degree (MD) has decreased given the ubiquitous need for postgraduate training to enable unsupervised practice.[114] For trainees interested in subspecialization, the length of postgraduate training has increased even further. While the MD reflects a uniform, broad qualification to practice, residencies and fellowships show a very large variety of medical qualifications. Specialties in the US have increased in number between 1960 and 2011 from 18 to 158.[115] While there is variation in the length of residencies and fellowships, the total training has become so lengthy that authors have called for a decrease in length by shortening compartments; authors have also called for a better justification for the multitude of subspecialties and the differences in number of specialties and length of programs between countries.[12,115]

It has been argued that more efficient training could decrease education costs, reduce educational debt, and permit physicians to enter practice at a younger age, thereby improving physician workforce supply.[13,116,117] Others have criticized the waste of time in the fourth year of medical school because of undue efforts in application for residency.[118] While a shortening in length of the continuum would hold for all trainees, Emanuel and Fuchs suggest an increased emphasis on individualized instruction and assessment of core competencies rather than on time served.[12] This is in concordance with the Carnegie Foundation Report recommendation that medical education should "provide options for individualizing the learning processes for students and residents, such as offering the possibility of fast tracking within and across levels."[119]

Box 4.1 Examples of TVMT within and across compartments

There are multiple examples of TVMT across the educational continuum. Since the turn of the century in Australia, students can either enter medical school directly from high school ("direct entry") or after obtaining a bachelor's degree ("graduate entry")[120]; other countries, such as the UK and the Netherlands have followed this model.[121,122]

The United States has combined premedical-medical school programs, and Canada has both three- and four-year medical schools. Three-year medical schools in the US, seeing short-lived initiatives in the 1970s, are again being developed. Some programs award all students an MD degree after three years and others only to select students.

The New York University (NYU) School of Medicine has a three-year MD program that offers conditional acceptance into postgraduate training programs within the institution. NYU also has an opt-in pathway were students can decide to fast track at the beginning of the third year of medical school and an opt-out pathway back to a 4-year program. Dutch medical schools are currently developing elective *dedicated transitional year* programs for final year students interested in a limited number of residency options with a shorter duration.

In addition to TVMT from premedical to medical school and medical school to residency, there are also examples of TVMT from residency to post-graduate training (e.g., the American Board of Internal Medicine fast-track research pathway – see http://www.abim.org/certification/ policies/research-pathway/policies-requirements.aspx.

The learning and training trajectory between secondary school and unsupervised clinical practice for individuals is usually about 14 years and consists of three to five distinct educational programs. As was highlighted in the section on history, the length of training is basically an arbitrary and historically and politically agreed upon entity that proved workable, but that currently has no empirical grounding.

The same holds for the compartments within this continuum. Within and between various countries, compartments may be combined, may include mandatory service years, and may have a different lengths.[123] Figure 4.1 shows two examples, with columns representing years.

Figure 4.1 Common program arrangement across the medical education continuum – two examples from North American and European countries

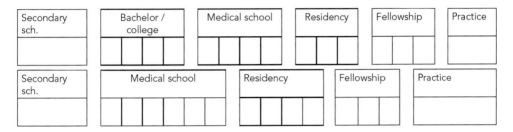

Time-variable medical training may be considered from the perspective of each of these components, separately or from the perspective of the continuum.

4.2 Time variability across compartments of the continuum

The path to unsupervised practice, as noted above, is characterized by multiple transitions between levels of training (undergraduate to graduate to postgraduate). Furthermore, these transitions are often characterized by relocation to new institutions. In many countries, oversight and regulation of UME is distinct from GME.[117] Time-variable medical training necessitates mutual agreement and understanding between program directors across the transition points regarding how "readiness" for progression is defined. The "givers" and "receivers" need to agree on definitions of competence and what level of skills is required or expected. There also must be robust assessment systems that assess trainee competence and transition readiness. This would require a "uniform set of milestones and competencies whereby assessment cuts across each level of medical school, residency, and fellowship, thus linking UME and GME as a continuum of learning."[117] This would require coordination within and across what are now silos of pre-medical education, UME, GME, and accrediting organizations.[117]

However, there is also a more local option. If UME and GME are both viewed as compartments of one program, then it is not unthinkable that a student moves to a residency within university or a university area. This has the benefit of opening opportunities for close, local collaboration between compartments, avoiding time- and effort-consuming application procedures for students, and providing possibilities of mutual evaluation of students and clinical environments to seek a local match and to transition at well-chosen moments. This would avoid the "July effect" of a sudden decrease in experienced residents for care provision in teaching hospitals in North America.[124,125] Though daunting, there are early demonstration projects of this coordinated approach (Box 4.2).

Box 4.2 Examples of programs connecting compartments the medical education continuum

The "Education in Pediatrics Across the Continuum" (EPAC) project (previously known as the Pediatrics Redesign Project) is a four-institution pilot (University of California, San Francisco; University of Colorado; University of Minnesota; and University of Utah) that tests the feasibility of using competencies and EPAs as the platform for variable time-based advancement across UME and GME for students who know they are interested in pediatrics.[126] Students enter the program in the second year of medical school and finish residency when they complete all the requirements.[127]

A somewhat diferent example is provided in the Josiah Macy Jr. Foundation supported "Accelerated Pathways" project that organizes three-year medical programs in North America. This may be viewed as a attempt to vary time in training for selected populations with the intention of connecting to selected residencies. Sudents for such pathways are selected at the beginning of medical school after the first year if they meet conditions of proficiency and interest to practice in certain regions and specialties (usually rural areas and primary care). Most of the nine schools that offer this option have longitudinal continuity clerkships and adapt the timing of medical licensing examinations. A key component of success is to engage students in a residency department where they will be placed after graduation to solidify their career choice. The samples are small but the students who accelerate reportedly meet the standards for graduation of four-year programs.[13,128]

4.3 Issues to consider with TVMT across continuum compartments

Even if there are models for how to have flexibility across the continuum, important caveats must be noted. First, there may be trainees ready for early transition from a competency perspective but who are yet not ready to commit to a particular specialty or subspecialty and will, therefore, require longer training. Programs will need to be flexible should a learner require time to gain the experiences that are felt necessary to make career decisions. It will be important to ensure that TVMT does not lead to premature career commitment and subsequent career choice mismatch or regret. On the other hand, some students may enter medical training with preferences that can be elaborated in electives during medical school, enabling earlier career choice. Anecdotal observations give the impression that students usually prefer to remain in training for a longer rather than shorter time period (OtC personal communication with senior medical students, 2005–2017). Drivers of this impression appear to be students' feeling prepared for practice and their perceived chances of being accepted in residency training. Critical for students are comparisons to peers caused by competitive applications for further career advancement.

Second, many authors describe how trainees in time-based programs are inadequately prepared to commence graduate medical training,[129,130] fellowship programs,[131] or unsupervised practice,[132] while Napolitano et al. report that young attendings may be more optimistic than senior surgeons.[133] For example, there are gaps between what residents have been documented as being able to do without supervision and what they can actually do without supervision. In fact, many undergraduate training programs have immersive transition courses (often called "boot camps"[134]) immediately prior to graduation to help prepare learners for transition. Similarly, many graduate training programs also have immersion experiences at the onset of graduate training. Time-variable medical training will either require trainees to be better prepared for transition or require flexibility in the timing of these transition experiences. Furthermore, it will be important to determine the degree to which a learner could be deemed competent but still lack the depth of clinical exposure, direct patient care experience, maturity, and leadership skills necessary for transition.[13]

Third, variable timing of finishing graduate training, either to enter practice or to transition to postgraduate fellowship training, can present significant workforce issues for institutions that rely on graduate and postgraduate trainees to deliver care using fixed schedules. There will likely be unpredictability of training start and end dates. Institutions would need to be nimble and flexible to meet workforce needs as trainees complete training early. Additionally, training programs would need to have flexibility to potentially accommodate more or fewer trainees at any given time, such as when an undergraduate trainee is ready to progress into graduate training faster than graduate trainees are competent to complete a program.

Along these lines, it will be important to ensure that there is congruence across transition points between programs participating in TVMT to assure availability of training spots. For example, if medical schools start TVMT, there must be enough graduate training programs that are willing to and can accept the undergraduate trainees from these programs. In the United States, there are ongoing discussions about consortia that will accept trainees from three-year programs with ability to share tracked learner data.[135]

Fourth, in some countries graduate and postgraduate training positions are acquired through a time-based process with single, fixed entry points for applications and position notifications (i.e., the National Residency Match Program). In a TVMT paradigm, how training positions are acquired would need to be revisited. Other countries offer transitions that are more flexible, such as the Dutch example (in Box 4.3), which shows how a system could accommodate temporary mismatches in numbers of graduates and available residency places.

Box 4.3 Transition from medical school to residency in The Netherlands

Dutch medical schools offer six-year programs (or shorter, graduate-entry programs for a minority of students). Students are scheduled in clinical rotations in years 4–6 (the 'master phase') and only a minority graduates exactly at the minimum time. On average, medical students take 6.5 to 7 years to graduate, and graduation ceremonies are held multiple times across the year. Students then apply in an open-market system for residency positions of their choice that also commence at different moments in the year.[136] Most medical graduates take time off after graduation (six months to a year or more) to work in healthcare settings, do research projects (including PhD training), assist in educational projects, or do something different, before they apply for residency. As residencies can start and conclude at various moments across the year and residency training positions are filled whenever vacant, flexible, individualized workplace curricula usually do not create workforce problems.

Fifth, communicating a trainee's skills and developing competence within and across programs will be even more important in a TVMT system. Portfolios of competence may be one approach. How much these portfolios require standardization in content and presentation would need to be decided. "Statements of Awarded Responsibility" (STARs) could be used to document summative entrustment decisions prior to transition or before completing training.[137,138] Models for how to effectively use portfolios for learner handoffs would need to be investigated, to evaluate how mentors can promote a longitudinal competency assessment across the UME-GME continuum. Learner assessment in TVMT is discussed in the next section.

5. THE NEED FOR COMPREHENSIVE LEARNER ASSESSMENT IN TIME-VARIABLE MEDICAL TRAINING

The concept of TVMT argues that, rather than specified time durations as a basis for making decisions about progress through a program, performance measures, as indicators of competence, are necessary. This basic principle of competency-based education has a number of implications for assessment.

5.1 The need for precision in assessment

One implication of competency-based education is the need for a clear distinction between assessment and the judgments and decisions that are made on those assessment data. Competency-based education emphasizes competencies and criteria for demonstrating competence. Decisions that need to be made, specifically higher stakes decisions (e.g., graduation, termination) require higher-quality assessment data than do more formative, low-stakes decisions (e.g., learner feedback, remediation). Fundamentally, TVMT requires trustworthy judgments by the profession of its own members, a "time" as a criterion is replaced by established competence. Assessment merely provides data for these judgments and is only a means to this greater end, not the end itself. The inherent uncertainty and imprecision of assessment in aiding these decisions must not be forgotten.

A related implication is that assessments should be diverse in methodology and in the outcomes assessed. Judgments about competence are complex and cannot be done with confidence on data that are unidimensional, regardless of how psychometrically sound they may be. The targets of assessment include the specified competencies for a program but also need to recognize that there are "implicit" components of professional development that may not be measurable. "Not everything that can be counted counts, and not everything that counts can be counted."* Competency decisions must also recognize that competence is more than the sum of the parts. Elemental assessments (e.g., checklists) may not capture the higher order relationships among the elements that constitute expert performance.

5.2 The need for more continuous and longitudinal assessment

Another implication is that, because competency decisions can be made at any time, assessment needs to be (more or less) continuous. This poses considerable demand on administrative and logistical resources. Furthermore, continuous assessment may blur the distinction for learners as to the purposes of the assessments—whether for high- or low-stakes purposes. This ambiguity may have a negative impact on the feedback culture of the program. Flexible scheduling of assessments becomes particularly challenging when large numbers of learners need to be accommodated or when the assessment decisions are high stakes.

---

* William Bruce Cameron. Informal Sociology, a casual introduction to sociological thinking. New York, NY: Random House; 1963.

Traditionally, high-stakes assessments have been rigidly scheduled. The increased flexibility required by TVMT of such assessment schedules will require significant organizational changes in the relevant examination bodies.

More frequent and higher quality assessment will require new resources of expertise in assessment, information management structures, decision-making systems (e.g., clinical competence committees), and the like. Reallocating resources in the face of overall budgetary constraints will be one of the major challenges to implementing TVMT. Coordinating diverse assessments into an overall system will also challenge administrators.[139] A good example of this is provided by the increasing use of "clinical competency committees" (or "entrustment committees," as Brown et al. recently suggested[140]) to collect, review, and synthesize assessment data and make competency decisions.[108] At present, many of these committees predominantly focus the discussion on learners who are at risk. There would be additional time and resources involved in expanding the scope of competency committee discussions to all learners. These committees are also likely to make increasing demands for more and higher quality assessment data to help them make their decisions.

The need for greater diversity in the targets and methods of assessment could spur innovation and experimentation in assessment methods and procedures for integrating and using the results for decision making. It will no longer be viable to depend almost exclusively on infrequent written or performance examinations and faculty evaluations of clinical performance. Instead, using a variety of established and more innovative assessment methods, TVMT will move us toward taking advantage of naturally occurring data that can be used for assessment. These include learner products (e.g., entries in an electronic health record), faculty judgments (e.g., mini-CEX, other observations, case-based discussions), administrative data (e.g., prior qualifications and tests, activities performed), team-based performance (e.g., based on multi-source feedback), and others that may not be presently thought of as "good enough" for assessment purposes when such assessment is limited to high stakes, summative decisions.

In principle, the notion of the EPA illustrates this point.[73] As a naturally occurring task (e.g., conducting a risk factor assessment for a health-maintenance examination), these professional activities can be both units of instruction, but also vehicles for assessing performance of the given task. Another assessment development will require the incorporation of patient-level data (dashboards, chart audits, etc.). Gathering these data and understanding how they should inform decision making about individual competence pose intriguing measurement and logistical challenges. Learning analytics may serve to support such decisions[141] and mobile technology may be used for the collection of data in the natural course of clinical actvities. Warm et al. showed how tracking almost 200 internal medicine residents over three years with 360,000 data points proved feasible.[142] The divide between formative and summative assessment with that many observations may blur. This may be justified, but may not always be felt this way among learners; documentation of suboptimal performance and its related feedback is a sensitive issue.

5.3 Context specificity of assessment

Doing more assessments in more settings about more outcomes will inevitably force assessors and decision makers to come to grips with the issue of context specificity, as described previously. There are multiple contexts in which trainees care for patients, and competence in one context does not indicate competence in other contexts. Enough assessments by enough observers of enough cases over enough contexts will need to be the ideal, but an ideal that will need to be tempered by reality. One promising direction of development, however, is the use of e-portfolios and mobile technology to capture natural encounters in the workplace to provide feedback, formative assessment, and summative decision of progress.[143]

However, the greatest variability in workplace-based assessment remains due to raters, not trainees. In many institutions and training programs, there is a lack of time, resources, and infrastructure for faculty development in rater training to decrease this variability. The object of such training should, however, not just be to equate raters. Expert opinion, sometimes viewed as "subjectivity," is increasingly considered valuable and even necessary to arrive at valid assessment of clinical trainees.[144] This is a new domain of investigation,[145] related in part to entrustment decision making.[73,146]

6. LEGISLATIVE, REGULATORY, AND OTHER SYSTEM FACTORS AFFECTING TRAINING DURATION

6.1 Time-variable training and clinical service provision

The needs of predictable clinical service scheduling are incompatible with complete time-flexibility in competency-based education. Clinical service systems must be able to provide appropriate levels of skilled provider expertise for a given level of patient demand and trainees constitute an essential part of the workforce. Scheduling such resources requires predictability, which fits well with a traditional time-based educational framework. In contrast, TVMT may embody unpredictability of trainee schedules and availability because they may have "tested out" of further training time—and thus, further clinical service. Scheduling procedures, coordinating professional schedules, and patient "throughput" all challenge the idea of individually customized learning durations.

There are, of course, ways to make predictable clinical scheduling and TVMT more compatible. One might be reducing activities that do not directly contribute to clinical care or education ("scut"). Another would be to temper the strong claims of TVMT (i.e., that the learner must move on to the next stage of training immediately upon demonstrating "competence.") Instead, individualized learning plans could be used so that staying "in place" for an additional span of time was seen to support learning that is relatively content independent (e.g., communication, leadership development), thus making time required to fulfill clinical service more educationally beneficial as highlighted in the rimmed box in Figure 2.4. To complement flexibility from the educational side, clinical scheduling could be done more flexibly by better matching clinical need with appropriate providers.

One specific aspect of time variablility is working hours restrictions in residency. In surgery and medicine, the strict enforcement of the 80-hour rule in the US has been challenged. Recent studies looking into the effects of a flexible application of this rule conclude that flexibility had no adverse effects on patient outcomes, satisfaction, overall well-being, and educational quality,[147] while there may be an effect on personal and family activities.[148] The studies stirred significant discussion,[147,149] one element of which is the autonomy as a professional virtue that should allow for flexibility of working hours to allow for attending to patients when they need attention, potentially in conflict with duty hour restrictions.[150] The studies led ACGME to change duty hour rules to allow more flexibility as of July 2017.

6.2   Time-variable training, accreditation, and licensure

Time-variable medical training is not compatible with current accreditation and licensure standards. The vast majority of accreditation systems are still based on time and require specified durations for various aspects of education. A shift to TVMT will require a comprehensive change on the parts of accrediting bodies to specify their standards and expectations in metrics that are not simply the passage of time. Quantification of outcomes, whether in the form of competencies or other frameworks, will require data and evidence that, in turn, require more explicit judgment about standards and the trustworthiness of the evidence. It remains to be seen how accrediting bodies will adapt; whether they will specify a uniform set of data/evidence or whether they will allow institutional diversity in the form of the evidence.

Arguably, accreditation and licensure should be malleable to fit TVMT. Adaptation would require flexibility on the part of authorized decision makers as well as significant revision of these policies and regulations. The transitions from medical school to postgraduate training and from postgraduate training to practice are two significant examples of the incompatibility. Flexibility in the time required for medical school may be of little value if the entrance to postgraduate training is restricted to one entry period per calendar year. Similarly, a graduated approach to professional licensure, as postgraduate trainees master various competencies but still need to work on others, will require major changes in the current model of all-or-nothing licenses.

There are some small-scale experiments that indicate the ways these regulatory structures could be reshaped. The Education in Pediatrics Across the Continuum (EPAC) project (previously known as the Pediatrics Redesign Project) is a pilot implementation of using competencies to build a bridge between medical school and residency, allowing medical students to enter residency at the same institution on the basis of attained competence rather than time.[127] However, this innovation has not explicitly dealt with the problem of clinical service and TVMT.

In countries in which there is not a structure dictating immediate transition from medical school to postgraduate training, learners have opportunities to accumulate clinical or research experience and be better equipped for a residency application. This structure creates time variability naturally, but the goals of these interim activities are often defined idiosyncratically rather than in reference to clearly defined competencies. Even though such systems are more compatible with time variability, they do not translate into formally recognized "credit" towards subsequent training. Rather, it is a variable interval between one stage of training and the next, with no formal tracking and accrediting of competencies that might have been acquired in this interval.

6.3 Time-variable training, credits, and tuition

Other institutional structures that fit poorly with TVMT include credit hours and tuition calculations that are based on educational activities of a fixed duration. TVMT calls into question what students are paying for with their tuition—a degree or a set amount of time within an academic setting with access to faculty and other educational opportunities. Should students pay the same tuition for a medical degree regardless of how long it takes them to demonstrate competence or should tuition be pro-rated by the duration of training? Many universities have an incentive structure that financially rewards the school for students who take longer to earn their degree and spend more in tuition. A change to a TVMT structure would, therefore, require a reconfiguration of the economic model of higher and health professions education.

These incompatibilities arise in part because of the differences between higher education, where competency-based education originated in the 1980s (see sections 5 and 6), and medical education, where it is currently being applied. There are important contrasts between the goals and intentions for competency-based education within higher education[*] and medical education. Whereas competency-based education in medicine is designed to define and assure professional competence, competency-based education in higher education (in some countries) is seen as a vehicle to reduce costs, to increase access to education for non-traditional students who can demonstrate competence gained through work or life experience as credit toward a degree,[**] and to tailor vocational training better to the demands of the labor market. The contrasting perspectives on compe tency-based education between higher and medical education should be kept in mind to avoid confusion when communicating to the public. They should also guide our careful adaptation of competency-based education to the medical education setting.

---

[*] American Institute for Research. Evaluation for Improvement: Making the Case for Competency-Based Education. http://www.air.org/resource/evaluation-improvement-making-case-competency-based-education. Accessed 11 January 2017.

[**] Public Agenda. Shared Design Elements and Emerging Practices of Competency-Based Education Programs. PUBLIC AGENDA: 2015. Available online at www.cbenetwork.org.

7. MANAGING EXPECTATIONS RELATED TO TIME VARIABILITY IN TRAINING

The nature of perceptions and experiences is highly affected by expectations. Experiences of visitors to a museum for example are more affected by variations in expectations than by variations in exhibitions.[151] Teacher expectations may affect learner development through self-fulfilling prophecy mechanisms.[152]

In education, the psychology of expectation can be used powerfully in dialogues with learners. From the moment of admission to medical school, learners face "high expectations" and many clinical evaluations use a "below/meets/exceeds expectations" framework for evaluation, feedback, and admonitions. Expectations can be considered a light version of a contract, including agreement concerning some form of exchange among two parties. A provider (e.g., educational institute or a teacher) expresses expectations as a condition for reward (e.g., a diploma), and the receiver expects to receive the reward if these expectations are met. Breaches of contracts cause pain and a sense of injustice or unfairness in at least one party.

Managing expectations can affect the motivation and emotion of experiences and the feeling of fairness in evaluation. Medical students may be prepared to invest substantial effort in studying if well-informed ahead, but may feel deeply disappointed if misinformed at an early stage. Setting adequate expectations provides learners with an important tool to control their near future planning.

Expectations in education can refer to several conditions, three of which are educational objectives, a sense of time and effort needed to meet expectations, and the consequences of failure to meet them. Expectations not only are set by an educational institution and teachers, but also may come from the self, peers, and the outside world (friends, family, future employers, society).

Time-variable medical training presents a disruption to existing expectations. Schools that enroll students in classes that are labeled with a year of graduation will face necessary explanations and possibly embarrassment if a student graduates a year later. A fixed length of graduate training may also have this effect. A program that offers time-variable training, moving to a less strict time expectation and a more strict standards expectation, faces a difficulty of communication. Meeting or not meeting the first expectation (less strict time expectation) is immediately visible to everyone, while the latter (more strict standards) is hardy visible to anyone.

7.1 Individual expectations

Moving from an existing training arrangement to a new format can cause anxiety among trainees. While several authors have advocated a shortening of the medical education continuum,[12,115] personal observation by the lead author of this paper (OtC) suggests residents generally are not fond of shortening training, afraid to have fewer opportunities to meet expectations (personal communication with residents over a prolonged time period). The possibility to start practice and accumulating income may counter this anxiety, but these considerations are fundamentally different.

Why is managing expectations for individual learners important in TVMT? If the paradigm is graduation when all standards are met, then all should feel, on average, equally confident. However, time is often considered an indicator of capability. Graduates from medical schools meeting standards in a shorter time may feel valued more and may expect to be prioritized earlier by residency programs in application procedures if "faster" is perceived as "smarter." However, the opposite may be true too. A student taking "longer" may be perceived as having "more experience." Specialists with a longer residency training *program* may thus expect to be regarded as more proficient. In other words in TVMT, short length of individual training when compared with peers in similar programs (by supervisors, by future employers, future residencies, or by themselves) may be equated with high individual quality, and a long length of training *program* with high collective quality.

Expectations for individuals may be manageable if a longer or shorter length is not perceived as a deviation from the majority's length. However, if completion of training is not planned at a fixed moment in the year, and the program can accommodate other reasons for time variability (notably, doing research and family building; see section 4 and box 4.2) then time variability may be liberated from competitive notions of time, speed, and proficiency. Trainees should finish education at a reasonable, but not fixed time. "Reasonable" has not been defined,[153] but clearly, a training period that is doubled or condensed to half, caused by variation in developmental progression, may no longer be considered reasonable. Variations may be thought of as not exceeding up to +/- 20% of the average individual time. Trainees who exceed +20% time may be considered to fall outside a reasonable zone, while trainees who complete training in shorter than

-20% of time, may be faced with detrimental consequences of lack of experience (see also the section on dwell time).*

Finally, individual expectations may be managed by a culture that embraces learning after training. Learners may graduate from medical school and/or residency with varying portfolios of acquired competencies and mastered EPAs if programs are based on core and elective EPAs. The prospect of acquiring the permission to execute additional EPAs in the future, after a period of supervision, may alleviate anxiety among learners. While this paper does not pertain to lifelong learning upon completing formal training, clearly health professionals will need to actively keep learning, particularly given the rapidly changing health care context. Part of professional work should be devoted to learning; consequently clinical service schedules need to accommodate that training.

7.2 Institutional expectations

Institutional expectations may relate to investments in education and the institutional status. It is in the institution's interest to graduate top-level trainees, to contain costs, and to attract superior trainees. Reducing tuition fees for learners who show a shorter training time may be beneficial to attract applicants from a wider pool, but may reduce revenue. And interestingly, the definition of "top-level" is not unambiguous, as previously illustrated.

There is a risk that institutions will advertise the average training length if it appears to be short and consequently push to *expect* a shorter training time, while some learners may require *more* time. In other words, if the most proficient learners become the standard, then the basic idea of time variability to allow all graduates to achieve standards comes under threat. This could put even great pressure on making sure programs select the very best talent that can perform in this environment.

7.3 Societal expectations

Society at large has expectations about training that are less explicit. Its primary concern is quality and safety of the health care system and competence of its health care workforce. It is likely that its regulatory bodies are more concerned with standards than with the time it takes individuals to meet these standards, and

---

*   We acknowledge that this is an arbitrary figure that should require investigation.

that time-variable training with this purpose would be welcomed. The definition of standards is not simple, and society at large must rely on professional bodies that certify physicians and specialists. These bodies, responsible for certification and recertification and for accreditation of educational programs, will need to accept time variability in training and be co-responsible for the maintenance of standards.

8. Coda

This document was written to shed light on the various aspects of TVMT. Rather than providing recommendations, it was intended to stimulate a well-informed discussion. Time-variable medical training is a multifaceted concept that is easily defendable as a logical consequence of competency-based education,[4–6] but its implications are manifold. Several elements are not yet well documented and should be studied more in depth. Potential topics and questions for a research agenda include, but are not limited to, the following:

- The analysis of what is a reasonable time for training to meet specified objectives of workplace learning. Until now, length of training has not been clearly justified with educational arguments and a detailed analysis of relevant factors may provide a better grounding of choices from durations.

- The relationship between duration of training; working hours per week; learning effect; and stress, burnout, and depression has not been studied well.

- Feasibility studies involving the combination of educational and health service perspectives

- Small-scale pilot experiments with time-variable training may be carried out, followed by larger feasibility and effect studies.

- Justifications of time variability to maintain standards will remain a substantive reasearch question.

- Studies to distinguish when repetition of experiences adds productively to the development of competence and when it becomes redundant.

- Studies of how different clinical contexts and team types can be used to strategically support trainee development.

Such educational studies are not easy. One reason is that both education and health care are complex adaptive systems that will react to any experimental intervention that is carried out for research purposes. Randomized trials may seem feasible for some questions,[148] but not for most. The medical education community must move forward in making decisions that appear needed and useful, and will have to rely on best evidence, practice experience, and logical reasoning, even if proof is not likely to become conclusive.

ACKNOWLEDGEMENTS

The authors thank the reviewers of this document, Dr. Catherine R. Lucey (University of California, San Francisco School of Medicine) and Dr. Robert A. Blouin (University of North Carolina-Chapel Hill), for very valuable comments on an earlier version of this manuscript.

REFERENCES

1. Frank JR, Mungroo R, Ahmad Y, et al. Toward a definition of competency-based education in medicine: a systematic review of published definitions. *Med Teach.* 2010;32(8):631–637.

2. Irby DM, Cooke M, O'Brien BC. Calls for reform of medical education by the Carnegy Foundation for the Advancement of Teaching: 1910 and 2010. *Acad Med.* 2010;85:220–227.

3. Jason H. Effective medical instruction: Requirements and possibilities. In: Van den Bussche R, Simpson M, editors. *Proceedings of a 1969 International Symposium on Medical Education.* Leuven, Belgium: Medica; 1970. p. 5–8.

4. McGaghie WC, Miller GE, Sajid AW, Telder TW. *Competency-based curriculum development in medical education - an introduction.* Chicago, Ill.: Center for Educational Development, University of Illinois at the Medical Center, Chicago, IL, USA and World Health Organization; 1978.

5. Long DM. Competency based residency training: the next advance in graduate medical education. *Acad Med.* 2000 Jan;75:1178–1183.

6. Carraccio C, Wolfsthal SD, Englander R, Ferentz K, Martin C. Shifting paradigms: from Flexner to competencies. *Acad Med.* 2002;77(5):361–367.

7. Carraccio C, Englander R, Van Melle E, et al. Advancing competency-based medical education: A charter for clinician-educators. *Acad Med.* 2016;91(5):645–649.

8. ten Cate O. Competency-based medical education and its competency frameworks. In: Mulder M, editor. *Competence-based Vocational and Professional Education: Bridging the Worlds of Work and Education.* Dordrecht, the Netherlands: Springer Science+Business Media BV; 2016.

9. Halsted WS. The training of the surgeon. *Johns Hopkins Hosp Bull.* 1904;(162):267–275.

10. European Economic Community. Council Directive 75/363/EEC concerning the coordination of provisions laid down by law, regulation or adminitrative action in respect to activities of doctors. *Off J Eur Communities.* 1975;(L):167/14-167/16.

11. European Parliament. Directive 2013/55/EU of the European Parliament and of the council of 20 November 2013 amending Directive 2005/36/EC on the recognition of professional qualifications and Regulation. Off J Eur Union [Internet]. 2013;(354):132–70. Available from: http://eur-lex.europa.eu/LexUriServ/LexUriServ.do?uri=OJ:L:2013:354:0132:0170:en:PDF

12. Emanuel EJ, Fuchs VR. Shortening medical training by 30%. *JAMA.* 2012;307(11):1143–1144.

13. Cangiarella J, Gillespie C, Shea JA, Morrison G, Abramson SB. Accelerating medical education: a survey of deans and program directors. *Med Educ Online.* 2016;21(31794):1–8.

14. Frank JR, Snell LS, ten Cate O, et al. Competency-based medical education: theory to practice. *Med Teach.* 2010;32(8):638–645.

15. Sonnadara RR, Mui C, McQueen S, et al. Reflections on competency-based education and training for surgical residents. *J Surg Educ.* 2014;71(1):151–158.

16. Nousiainen MT, Mcqueen SA. Simulation for teaching orthopaedic residents in a competency- based curriculum: Do the benefits justify the increased costs ? *Clin Orthop Relat Res.* 2016;474(4):935–944.

17. Sonnadara RR, Vliet A Van, Safir O, Alman B. Orthopedic boot camp: Examining the effectiveness of an intensive surgical skills course. *Surgery.* 2011;149(6):745–749.

18. Goldberg C, Insel PA. Preparing MD-PhD students for clinical rotations. *Acad Med.* 2013;88(6):745–747.

19. DeLuca GC, Ovseiko P V, Buchan AM. Personalized medical education: Reappraising clinician-scientist training. *Sci Transl Med.* 2016;8(321):321fs21-3.

20. Blair JE, Mayer AP, Caubet SL, Norby SM, O'Connor MI, Hayes SN. Pregnancy and parental leave during graduate medical education. *Acad Med.* 2016;91(7):972–978.

21. Mayer AP, Blair JE, Ko MG, et al. Gender distribution of U.S. medical school faculty by academic track type. *Acad Med.* 2014;89(2):312–317.

22. Rich A, Viney R, Needleman S, Griffin A, Woolf K. "You can't be a person and a doctor': the work-life balance of doctors in training-a qualitative study. *BMJ Open.* 2016;6(12):e013897.

23. Mata DA, Ramos MA, Bansai N, et al. Prevalence of depression and depressive symptoms among resident physicians: A systematic review and meta-analysis. *JAMA.* 2015;314(22):2373–2383.

24. Rotenstein LS, Ramos MA, Torre M, et al. Prevalence of depression, depressive symptoms, and suicidal ideation among medical students: A systematic review and meta-analysis. *JAMA.* 2016;316(21):2214–2236.

25. Billett S. Mimetic learning at work: Learning in the circumstances of practice. 1st ed. Dordrecht: Springer; 2014.

26. Tyler RW. Basic Principles of Curriculum and Instruction. Chicago: University of Chicago Press; 1949.

27. Bloom B, Engelhart M, Furst E, Hill W, Krathwohl D. Taxonomy of educational objectives: the classification of educational goals; Handbook I: Cognitive Domain. New York, NY: Longmans, Green; 1956.

28. Krathwohl DR, Bloom BS, Masia BB. Taxonomy of Educational Objectives, the Classification of Educational Goals. Handbook II: Affective Domain. New York, NY: David McKay Co, Inc; 1973.

29. Chan BY. After Tyler, what? A current issue in curriculum theory. *Educ J.* 1977;6(1):21–31.

30. Carroll JB. A model of school learning. *Teach Coll Rec.* 1963;64:723–733.

31. Carroll JB. The Carroll Model - A 25-year retrospective and prospective view. *Educ Res.* 1989;18(1):26–31.

32. Bloom BS. Learning for mastery. *Instruction and Curriculum.* 1968;1(2):1–11.

33. McGaghie WC. Mastery learning: It is time for medical education to join the 21st century. *Acad Med* 2015;90(11):1–4.

34. Kulik C-LC, Kulik JA, Bangert-Drowns RL. Effectiveness of mastery learning programs: a meta-analysis. *Rev Educ Res.* 1990;60(2):265–299.

35. Schunk DH. Learning Theories. An Educational Perspective. 6th ed. Schunk DH, editor. Boston: Pearson Education Inc., Boston; 2012. 1-561 p.

36. Lineberry M, Soo Park Y, Cook DA, Yudkowsky R. Making the case for mastery learning assessments: Key issues in validation and justification. *Acad Med* [Internet]. 2015;90(11):1145–1150. Available from: http://content.wkhealth.com/linkback/openurl?sid=WKPTLP:landingpage&an=00001888-900000000-98712

37. Yudkowsky R, Park YS, Lineberry M, Knox A, Ritter EM. Setting mastery learning standards. *Acad Med* [Internet]. 2015;90(11):1495–1500. Available from: http://content.wkhealth.com/linkback/openurl?sid=WKPTLP:landingpage&an=00001888-900000000-98690

38. Motola I, Devine LA, Chung HS, Sullivan JE, Issenberg SB. Simulation in healthcare education: a best evidence practical guide. AMEE Guide No. 82. *Med Teach.* 2013;35(10):e1511-e1530.

39. McGaghie WC, Issenberg SB, Cohen ER, Barsuk JH, Wayne DB. Does simulation-based medical education with deliberate practice yield better results than traditional clinical education? A meta-analytic comparative review of the evidence. *Acad Med.* 2011;86(6):706–711.

40. Macnamara BN, Hambrick DZ, Oswald FL. Deliberate practice and performance in music, games, sports, education, and professions: A meta-analysis. *Psychol Sci.* 2014;24(8):1608–1618.

41. van de Wiel MWJ, Van den Bossche P, Janssen S, Jossberger H. Exploring deliberate practice in medicine: how do physicians learn in the workplace? *Adv Health Sci Educ Theory Pract.* 2011;16(1):81–95.

42. Chung J Il, Kim N, Um MS, et al. Learning curves for colonoscopy: A prospective evaluation of gastroenterology fellows at a single center. *Gut Liver.* 2010;4(1):31–35.

43. ten Cate O. The false dichotomy of quality and quantity in the discourse around assessment in competency-based education. *Adv Heal Sci Educ.* 2014;20(3):835–838.

44. Pusic M V, Boutis K, Hatala R, Cook DA. Learning curves in health professions education. *Acad Med.* 2015;90(8):1034–1042.

45. Ravesloot C, van der Schaaf M, Haaring C, et al. Construct validation of progress testing to measure knowledge and visual skills in radiology. *Med Teach.* 2012;34(12):1047–1055.

46. Maquet P. The role of sleep in learning and memory. *Science.* 2001;294(5544):1048–1052 .

47. Kuriyama K, Stickgold R, Walker M. Sleep-dependent learning and motor-skill complexity. *Learn {&} Mem.* 2004;11(6):705–713.

48. Fogel SM, Ray LB, Binnie L, Owen AM. How to become an expert: A new perspective on the role of sleep in the mastery of procedural skills. *Neurobiol Learn Mem.* 2015;125:236–248.

49. Diekelmann S, Born J. The memory function of sleep. *Nat Rev Neurosci.* 2010;11(2):114–126.

50. Cepeda NJ, Pashler H, Vul E, Wixted JT, Rohrer D. Distributed practice in verbal recall tasks: A review and quantitative synthesis. *Psychol Bull.* 2006;132(3):354–380.

51. Kang SHK. Spaced repetition promotes efficient and effective learning: Policy implications for instruction. *Policy Insights from Behav Brain Sci.* 2016;3(1):12–19.

52. Kapler I V., Weston T, Wiseheart M. Spacing in a simulated undergraduate classroom: Long-term benefits for factual and higher-level learning. *Learn Instr.* 2015;36:38–45.

53. Gerbier E, Toppino TC. The effect of distributed practice: Neuroscience, cognition, and education. *Trends Neurosci Educ.* Elsevier; 2015;4(3):49–59.

54. Mega C, Ronconi L, De Beni R. What makes a good student? How emotions, self-regulated learning, and motivation contribute to academic achievement. *J Educ Psychol.* 2014;106(1):121–131.

55. Kusurkar RA, ten Cate TJ, van Asperen M, Croiset G. Motivation as an independent and a dependent variable in medical education: a review of the literature. *Med Teach.* 2011;33(5):e242-e262.

56. Dweck CS. Self-theories: Their role in motivation, personality, and development. Philadelphia: Psychology Press; 1999.

57. Teunissen PW, Bok HGJ. Believing is seeing: how people's beliefs influence goals, emotions and behaviour. *Med Educ.* 2013;47(11):1064–1072.

58. Ericsson KA. Deliberate Practice and the Acquisition and Maintenance of Expert Performance in Medicine and Related Domains. *Acad Med.* 2004;79(10):S70–S81.

59. ten Cate TJ, Kusurkar RA, Williams GC. How self-determination theory can assist our understanding of the teaching and learning processes in medical education. AMEE guide No. 59. *Med Teach.* 2011;33(12):961–973.

60. ten Cate O. Entrustability of professional activities and competency-based training. *Med Educ.* 2005 Dec;39(12):1176–1177.

61. ten Cate O, Chen HC, Hoff RG, Peters H, Bok H, van der Schaaf M. Curriculum development for the workplace using entrustable professional activities (EPAs): AMEE Guide No. 99. *Med Teach.* 2015;37(12):983–1002.

62. Halpern SD, Detsky AS. Graded autonomy in medical education — Managing things that go bump in the night. *N Engl J Med.* 2014;370(12):1086–1089.

63. Fisher JF. Permanent resident. *Med Educ Online* [Internet]. 2016;21(31160):1–4. Available from: http://www.med-ed-online.net/index.php/meo/article/view/31160

64. ten Cate O. AM Last Page: What entrustable professional activities add to a competency-based curriculum. *Acad Med.* 2014;89(4):691.

65. Wiersma F, Berkvens J, ten Cate O. Flexibility in Individualized competency-based training with EPAs: Analyzing four cohorts of physician assistants in training. *Med Teach.* 2017; 39(5):535–539.

66. Touchie C, ten Cate O. The promise, perils, problems and progress of competency-based medical education. *Med Educ.* 2016;50(1):93–100.

67. Englander R, Flynn T, Call S, Carraccio C, Cleary L, Fulton TB, et al. Toward defining the foundation of the MD degree: Core entrustable professional activities for entering residency. *Acad Med.* 2016;91(10):1352–1358.

68. Touchie C, Boucher A, editors. Entrustable professional activities for the transition from medical school to residency. Ottawa, Ontario, Canada: Association of Faculties of Medicine of Canada; 2016.

69. Carraccio C, Englander R, Gilhooly J, et al. Building a Framework of Entrustable Professional Activities, Supported by Competencies and Milestones, to Bridge the Educational Continuum. *Acad Med.* 2017;92(3): 324–330.

70. Cruess RL, Cruess SR, Boudreau JD, Snell L, Steinert Y. Reframing medical education to support professional identity formation. *Acad Med.* 2014;89(11):1446–1451.

71. Hafferty F. Professionalism and the socialization of medical students. In: Cruess RL, Cruess SR, Steinert Y, editors. *Teaching Medical Professionalism.* Cambridge UK: Cambridge University Press; 2009. p. 53–73.

72. Jarvis-Selinger S, Pratt DD, Regehr G. Competency is not enough : Integrating identity formation into the medical education discourse. *Acad Med.* 2012;87(9):1185–1190.

73. ten Cate O, Hart D, Ankel F, Busari J, Englander R, Glasgow N, et al. Entrustment decision making in clinical training. *Acad Med.* 2016;91(2): 191–198.

74. Chen HC, Teherani A. Workplace affordances to increase learner engagement in the clinical workplace. *Med Educ.* 2015;49(12):1184–1186.

75. Norman G. Research in clinical reasoning: past history and current trends. *Med Educ.* 2005;39(4):418–427.

76. Custers EJFM. Thirty years of illness scripts: Theoretical origins and practical applications. *Med Teach.* 2015;37(5):457–462.

77. Hafler JP, Ownby AR, Thompson BM, et al. Decoding the learning environment of medical education: a hidden curriculum perspective for faculty development. *Acad Med* [Internet]. 2011 Apr [cited 2012 Mar 9];86(4):440–4. Available from: http://www.ncbi.nlm.nih.gov/pubmed/21346498

78. Hafferty F, Hafler J. The Hidden Curriculum, Structural Disconnects, and the Socialization of New Professionals. In: Hafler JP, editor. *Extraordinary Learning in the Workplace.* 1st ed. Dordrecht, the Netherlands: Springer Science+Business Media BV; 2011. p. 17–35.

79. Asch DA, Nicholson S, Srinivas SK, Herrin J, Epstein AJ. How do you deliver a good obstetrician? Outcome-based evaluation of medical education. *Acad Med.* 2014;89(1):24–26.

80. Asch DA, Nicholson S, Srinivas S, Herrin J, Epstein AJ. Evaluating obstetrical residency programs using patient outcomes. *JAMA.* 2009;302(12):1277–1283.

81. Lingard L, Sue-Chue-Lam C, Tait GR, et al. Pulling together and pulling apart: influences of convergence and divergence on distributed healthcare teams. *Adv Health Sci Educ Theory Pract.* 2017;22(5):1085–1099.

82. Hodges BD, Lingard L. The question of competence : reconsidering medical education in the twenty-first century. Hodges BD, Lingard L, editors. Ithaca, NY: Cornell University Press; 2012. 219 p.

83. Westerman M, Teunissen PW, van der Vleuten CPM, et al. Understanding the transition from resident to attending physician: a transdisciplinary, qualitative study. *Acad Med.* 2010;85(12):1914–1919.

84. Bernabeo EC, Holtman MC, Ginsburg S, Rosenbaum JR, Holmboe ES. Lost in transition: The experience and impact of frequent changes in the inpatient learning environment. *Acad Med.* 2011;86(5):591–598.

85. Worley P, Prideaux D, Strasser R, March R, Worley E. What do medical students actually do on clinical rotations? *Med Teach.* 2004;26(7):594–598.

86. Dornan T, Tan N, Boshuizen H, et al. How and what do medical students learn in clerkships? Experience based learning (ExBL). *Adv Health Sci Educ Theory Pract.* 2014;19(5):721–749

87. Park YS, Hodges BD, Tekian A. Evaluating the paradigm shift from time-based toward competency-based medical education: implications for curriculum and assessment. In: Wimmers PF, Mentkowski M, editors. *Assessing Competence in Professional Performance across Disciplines and Professions.* 1st ed. Springer International Publishing Switzerland; 2016. p. 411–425.

88. Holmboe E, Ginsburg S, Bernabeo E. The rotational approach to medical education: time to confront our assumptions? *Med Educ.* 2011;45(1):69–80.

89. Hirsh D, Ogur B, Thibault GE, Cox M. "Continuity" as an organizing principle for clinical education reform. *N Engl J Med.* 2007;356(8):858–866.

90. Bowen JL, Hirsh D, Aagaard E, et al. Advancing Educational Continuity in Primary Care Residencies. *Acad Med.* 2015;90(5):587–593.

91. Hudson JN, Poncelet AN, Weston KM, Bushnell JA, A Farmer E. Longitudinal integrated clerkships. *Med Teach.* 2016;39(1):7–13.

92. Ellman M, Tobin DG, Stepczynski J, Doolitttle B. Continuity of care as an educational goal but failed reality in resident training: Time to innovate. *J Grad Med Educ.* 2016;8(2):150–153.

93. Hirsh DA, Holmboe ES, ten Cate O. Time to trust: Longitudinal integrated clerkships and entrustable professional activities. *Acad Med.* 2013;89(2):201–204.

94. Hauer KE, ten Cate O, Boscardin C, Irby DM, Iobst W, O'Sullivan PS. Understanding trust as an essential element of trainee supervision and learning in the workplace. *Adv Health Sci Educ Theory Pract.* 2014;19(3):435–456.

95. Mylopoulos M, Brydges R, Woods NN, Manzone J, Schwartz DL. Preparation for future learning: A missing competency in health professions education? *Med Educ.* 2016;50(1):115–123.

96. ten Cate O, Billett S. Competency-based medical education: origins, perspectives and potentialities. *Med Educ.* 2014;48(3):325–332.

97. Pulakos ED, Arad S, Donovan MA, Plamondon KE. Adaptability in the workplace: development of a taxonomy of adaptive performance. *J Appl Psychol.* 2000;85(4):612–624.

98. Bates J, Ellaway RH. Mapping the dark matter of context: a conceptual scoping review. *Med Educ.* 2016;50(8):807–816.

99. Teunissen PW. Experience, trajectories, and reifications: An emerging framework of practice-based learning in healthcare workplaces. *Adv Health Sci Educ Theory Pract.* 2015 Oct;20(4):843–856.

100. Sfard A. On two metaphors for learning and the dangers of choosing just one. *Educ Res.* 1998;27(2):4–13.

101. Dornan T, Boshuizen H, King N, Scherpbier A. Experience-based learning: A model linking the processes and outcomes of medical students' workplace learning. *Med Educ.* Hope Hospital, School of Medicine, University of Manchester, Manchester, UK; 2007;41(1):84–91.

102. ten Cate O, Snell L, Carraccio C. Medical competence: The interplay between individual ability and the health care environment. *Med Teach.* 2010;32(8):669–675.

103. Mann K, Dornan T, Teunissen PW. Perspectives on learning. In: Dornan T, Mann K, Scherpbier A, Spencer J, editors. *Medical Education, Theory and Practice.* Edinburgh: Churchill-Livingstone; 2010. p. 11–38.

104. Wenger E. Conceptual tools for CoPs as social learning systems: Boundaries, identity, trajectories and participation. In: Blackmore C, editor. *Social Learning Systems and Communities of Practice*. London, UK: Springer London; 2010. p. 125–144.

105. Bleakley A, Bligh J, Browne J. Place matters : Location in medical education. In: *Medical Education for the Future: Identity, Power and Location*. 2011. p. 135–152.

106. Morcke AM, Dornan T, Eika B. Outcome (competency) based education: An exploration of its origins, theoretical basis, and empirical evidence. *Adv Health Sci Educ Theory Pract*. 2013;18(4):851–863.

107. Pangaro L, ten Cate O. Frameworks for learner assessment in medicine: AMEE Guide No. 78. *Med Teach*. 2013;35(6):e1197-e1210.

108. Hauer KE, Chesluk B, Iobst W, et al. Reviewing residents' competence: A qualitative study of the role of clinical competency committees in performace assessment. *Acad Med*. 2015;90(8):1084–1092.

109. Iobst WF, Sherbino J, ten Cate O, et al. Competency-based medical education in postgraduate medical education. *Med Teach*. 2010;32(8):651–656.

110. Hodges BD. A tea-steeping or i-Doc model for medical education? *Acad Med*. 2010;85(9 Suppl):S34-S44.

111. Luu S, Patel P, St-Martin L, et al. Waking up the next morning: Surgeons' emotional reactions to adverse events. *Med Educ*. 2012;46(12):1179–1188.

112. Dyrbye L, Shanafelt T. A narrative review on burnout experienced by medical students and residents. *Med Educ*. 2016;50(1):132–149.

113. Hashimoto DA, Bynum WE, Lillemoe KD, Sachdeva AK. See more, do more, teach more. *Acad Med*. 2016;91(6):757–760.

114. ten Cate O. What is a 21st-century doctor? Rethinking the significance of the medical degree. *Acad Med*. 2014;89(7):966–969.

115. Detsky AS, Gauthier SR, Fuchs VR. Specialization in medicine - How much is appropriate? *JAMA*. 2012;307(5):463–464.

116. Bleker OP, Blijham GH. Too Old, Too Smart and Too Expensive [Te oud, te knap en te duur]. *Med Contact* (Bussum). 1999;54(36):1201–1203.

117. Abramson SB, Jacob D, Rosenfeld M, et al. A 3-Year M.D. — Accelerating careers, diminishing debt. *N Engl J Med*. 2013;369(12):1085–1087.

118. Aagaard EM, Abaza M. The residency application process - Burden and consequences. *N Engl J Med*. 2016;374(4):301–303.

119. Cooke M, Irby D, O'Brien BC. Educating Physicians - A Call for Reform of Medical School and Residency. Hoboken, NJ, USA: Jossey-Bass/Carnegie Foundation for the Advancement of Teaching; Sep, 2010.

120. Finucane P, Nicholas T, Prideaux D, Finucane P, Nicholas T, Prideaux D. The new medical curriculum at Flinders University, South Australia: from concept to reality. *Med Teach.* 2001;23(1):76–79.

121. Cohen-Schotanus J, Schönrock-Adema J, Bouwkamp-Timmer T, van Scheltinga GRT, Kuks JBM. One-year transitional programme increases knowledge to level sufficient for entry into the fourth year of the medical curriculum. *Med Teach.* 2008;30(1):62–66.

122. ten Cate O. Medical education in the Netherlands. *Med Teach.* 2007;29(8):752–757.

123. Wijnen-Meijer M, Burdick W, Alofs L, Burgers C, ten Cate O. Stages and transitions in medical education around the world: clarifying structures and terminology. *Med Teach.* 2013;35(4):301–307.

124. Phillips DP, Barker GEC. A July spike in fatal medication errors: A possible effect of new medical residents. *J Gen Intern Med.* 2010;25(8):774–779.

125. Young JQ, Ranji SR, Wachter RM, Lee CM, Niehaus B, Auerbach AD. "July Effect": Impact of the Academic Year-End Changeover on Patient Outcomes. *Ann Intern Med.* 2011;155:309–315.

126. Aschenbrener CA, Ast C, Kirch DG. Graduate Medical Education: Its Role in Achieving a True Medical Education Continuum. *Acad Med.* 2015;90: Early Online.

127. Powell DE, Carraccio C, Aschenbrener CA. Pediatrics redesign project: a pilot implementing competency-based education across the continuum. *Acad Med.* 2011;86(11):e13.

128. Cangiarella J, Fancher T, Jones B, Dodson L, Leong SL, Hunsaker M, et al. Three-year MD programs: Perspectives from the Consortium of Accelerated Medical Pathway Programs (CAMPP). *Acad Med.* 2017;92(4):483–490.

129. Minter RM, Amos KD, Bentz ML, et al. Transition to Surgical Residency: A Multi-Institutional Study of Perceived Intern Preparedness and the Effect of a Formal Residency Preparatory Course in the Fourth Year of Medical School. *Acad Med.* 2015;90(8):1116–1124.

130. Raymond MR, Mee J, King A, Haist SA, Winward ML. What new residents do during their initial months of training. *Acad Med.* 2011;86(10 Suppl):S59-S62.

131. Mattar SG, Alseidi AA, Jones DB, et al. General surgery residency inadequately prepares trainees for fellowship: results of a survey of fellowship program directors. *Ann Surg*. 2013;258(3):440–449.

132. Soper NJ, DaRosa DA. Presidential address: Engendering operative autonomy in surgical training. *Surgery*. 2014;156(4):745–751.

133. Napolitano LM, Savarise M, Paramo JC, et al. Education: Are general surgery residents ready to practice? A survey of the American College of Surgeons Board of Governors and Young Fellows Association. *J Am Coll Surg*. 2014;218:1063–1072.e31.

134. Cohen ER, Barsuk JH, Moazed F, et al. Making July safer: Simulation-based mastery learning during intern boot camp. *Acad Med*. 2013;88(2):233–239.

135. Raymond JR, Kerschner JE, Hueston WJ, Maurana CA. The Merits and Challenges of Three-Year Medical School Curricula: Time for an Evidence-Based Discussion. *Acad Med*. 2015;90(10):1318–1323.

136. ten Cate O. Entrustment Decisions: Bringing the Patient into the Assessment Equation. *Acad Med*. 2017;92(6):736–738.

137. ten Cate O, Scheele F. Competency-based postgraduate training: Can we bridge the gap between theory and clinical practice? *Acad Med*. 2007;82(6):542–547.

138. ten Cate O. Entrustment as assessment: Recognizing the ability, the right and the duty to act. *J Grad Med Educ*. 2016;8(2):261–262.

139. van der Vleuten CPM, Schuwirth LWT, et al. A model for programmatic assessment fit for purpose. *Med Teach*. 2012;34(3):205–214.

140. Brown DR, Warren JB, Hyderi A, et al. Finding a path to entrustment in undergraduate medical education: A progress report from the AAMC Core Entrustable Professional Activities for Entering Residency Entrustment Concept Group. *Acad Med*. 2017;92(6):774–779.

141. van der Schaaf M, Donkers J, Slof B, et al. Improving workplace-based assessment and feedback by an E-portfolio enhanced with learning analytics. *Educ Technol Res Dev*. 2016;65:359–380.

142. Warm EJ, Held JD, Hellmann M, et al. Entrusting Observable Practice Activities and Milestones Over the 36 Months of an Internal Medicine Residency. *Acad Med*. 2016;91(10):1398.

143. Jonker G, Hoff RG, ten Cate OT. A case for competency-based anaesthesiology training with entrustable professional activities: An agenda for development and research. *Eur J Anaesthesiol*. 2015;32(2):71–76.

144. Gingerich A, Kogan J, Yeates P, Govaerts M, Holmboe E. Seeing the "black box" differently: assessor cognition from three research perspectives. *Med Educ*. 2014;48(11):1055–1068.

145. Gingerich A, Regehr G, Eva KW. Rater-based assessments as social judgments: rethinking the etiology of rater errors. *Acad Med*. 2011;86 (10 Suppl):S1-S7.

146. Damodaran A, Shulruf B, Jones P. Trust and risk: A model for medical education. *Med Educ*. 2017;51(9):892–902.

147. Asch DA, Bilimoria KY, Desai SV. Resident duty hours and medical education policy — Raising the evidence bar. *N Engl J Med*. 2017;376(18):1704–1706.

148. Bilimoria KY, Chung JW, Hedges LV, et al. National cluster-randomized trial of duty-hour flexibility in surgical training. *N Engl J Med*. 2016;374(8):713–727.

149. Correspondence. Surgical resident duty hours. *N Engl J Med*. 2016;374(24):1386–1388.

150. Rosenbaum L. Leaping without looking — Duty hours, autonomy, and the risks of research and practice. *N Engl J Med*. 2016;374:701–703.

151. Pekarik A, Schreiber J. The power of expectation. *Curator Museum J*. 2012;55(4):487–496.

152. Jussim L, Harber KD. Teacher expectations and self-fulfilling prophecies: Knowns and unknowns, resolved and unresolved controversies. *Personal Soc Psychol Rev*. 2005;9(2):131–155.

153. Maman-Dogma J, Rousseau M, Dove M, Rodriguez C, Meterissian S. Length of training in postgraduate medical education in Canada. Ottawa, Ontario, Canada: The Association of Faculties of Medicine of Canada; The College of Family Physicians of Canada; Le Collège des médecins du Québec; The Royal College of Physicians and Surgeons of Canada; 2011.

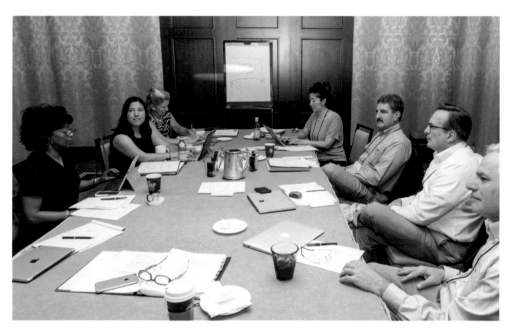

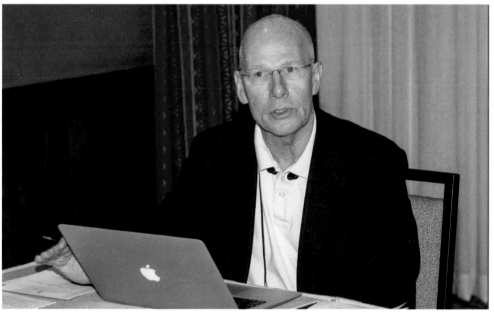

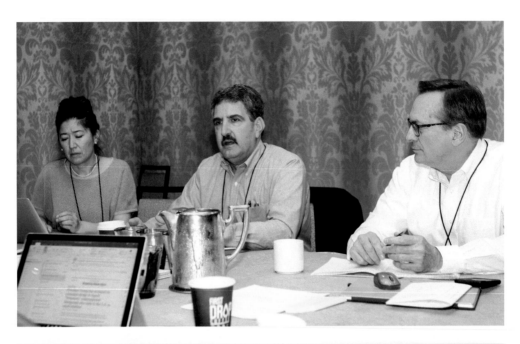

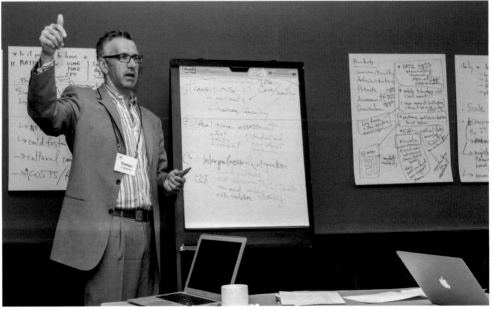

GREAT EXPECTATIONS:
COMPETENCY-BASED MEDICAL EDUCATION FROM REALITY TO VISION

Commissioned Paper

Damon Dagnone, MD, MMEd
CBME Faculty Lead, Postgraduate Medical Education
Associate Professor of Emergency Medicine
Faculty of Health Sciences
Queen's University, Canada

Denise Stockley, PhD
Professor and Scholar in Higher Education
Office of the Provost (Teaching and Learning Portfolio)
and the Faculty of Health Sciences
Queen's University, Canada

Leslie Flynn, MD, MEd
Vice-Dean, Education, Faculty of Health Sciences
Associate Professor, Departments of Psychiatry and Family Medicine
Queen's University, Canada
Clinician Educator, Royal College of Physicians & Surgeons of Canada

Richard Reznick, MD, MEd
Professor of Surgery
Dean, Faculty of Health Sciences
Queen's University, Canada

A VISION FOR THE FUTURE

Jane Miller applied to medical school when she was 21 years old, after completing a dual degree in a combined life sciences & humanities program. Her successful application process involved three stages of competency assessment: a one-month observership and group learning experience at her local university hospital under the supervision of a physician, clinical nurse, and a patient advocate; a multi-source assessment based on communication skills modules, knowledge base, and independent problem solving competency testing; and a third stage of long essay writing, reflections on her hospital experience, and in-person interviews with community members, physician supervisors, and other health care providers.

At the beginning of Jane's 2nd year of medical school, it was obvious from her electronic portfolio profile that she was clearly on a learning trajectory above that of her peers. The undergraduate medical education (UGME) committee approached her to enter an accelerated path to residency training in her chosen specialty, general internal medicine (GIM). Jane entered a more focused and intensive 12-month period to obtain the prerequisite competencies required for a successful transition to her graduate medical training.

Jane was accepted to the GIM program at her university center and took 36 months to complete her specialty certification training, which was within one standard deviation of all GIM trainees across the nation (based on a national electronic database updated annually). To facilitate her training, a faculty GIM mentor met with Jane quarterly to assist her with tracking her individual performance targets throughout her program. From the outset of her GIM training, she was assessed across a programmatic framework that included peer assessment, faculty supervisor assessment, multi-source team feedback, and direct patient and family feedback.

Throughout her residency training, she excelled in many areas and was in the 99th percentile in achieving numerous procedural skills and team-based competencies across care areas (inpatient, outpatient, emergency department, etc.). She was also nominated for an award for outstanding patient- and family-centered care in oncology. In other areas, however, she struggled and was in the 60% percentile in certain subspecialty area competencies, particularly in the medical expert and core knowledge milestones within nephrology and infectious diseases. To help her achieve these milestones, her faculty mentor/advisor helped design an individualized learning plan to create additional opportunities for repeat exposures and success in these domains.

Jane completed her specialty exams within the expected time frame, but delayed her final stage of residency training to take a two-month leave to get married. Six months later, Jane completed all GIM competencies required for her independent transition to practice, was given full certification by her accrediting body, and chose her first continuing professional development (CPD) faculty mentor. This mentor would meet with her bi-annually and assist with the development and implementation of an individualized continuing medical education strategy. Upon completion of her first five years of practice, she had the option to change her mentor and reduce her meetings to once annually throughout her career.

Jane began her career working at a large community hospital. She worked full-time as a clinician, and as per the certification standard for her speciality, she catalogued her patient encounters to demonstrate her exposure to the full breadth and depth of GIM and participated in quarterly simulation skills training days at her university training center. During the first year, these continuing professional development workshop days focused on a combination of procedural competencies on partial task trainers, team leader acute care/resuscitation competencies using high-fidelity, simulation-based resuscitation suites, and formal debriefing of critical events for interprofessional teams.

After three years working as a GIM physician, Jane re-entered training via a combined work/study program in oncology at her regional university teaching hospital three days a week, and continued to work two clinical days a week at her local community hospital. Jane's tuition for this training program was paid for by a governmental bursary program focused on enhancing clinical competencies. It was an appealing program because of its flexible training schedule, multidisciplinary approach, and cross-disciplinary training of individual and shared competencies. Jane was joined in her university multi-disciplinary training program by a number of health care professionals from many different hospitals and health centers within her region. These included nurses, pharmacists, surgeons, nurse practitioners, physiotherapists, occupational therapists, and family physicians—each of whom had various levels of training and experience.

During the 18 months of the oncology training program, Jane trained alongside her multi-disciplinary colleagues, achieving competencies in patient- and family-centered communication skills, medical and radiation oncology medicine, pharmaceutical sciences, surgical assist procedures, rehabilitation therapy, and nursing care. As well, she participated in a number of team-based simulation and reanimated resuscitative scenarios with expert critical care professionals to achieve competencies in acute care. Taking advantage of the research infrastructure available, Jane began her research career with a high-level journal publication of a novel multi-center research project examining the use of 'Fitbit physiological monitoring' for the creation of home-based algorithmic care pathways (using micro-dose polypharmacy pumps) based on daily variations in autonomous tracking of vital signs, subcutaneous blood work, and sleep-rest cycles. At the completion of her work/study program, Jane was offered the position of assistant director of the patient-centered community cancer care program for her region and spent the next decades thriving in numerous leadership roles.

BREAKDOWNS LEAD TO BREAKTHROUGHS – IMPERATIVES FOR CHANGE

Changes are happening in medical education that are shaking up the way we think about training health care professionals. Our current understanding of medical training has been focused on time on task, or what Snell and Frank[1] refer to as the "tea bag model." As physicians in training move through their rotations, there has been an assumption that when they finish, they will have achieved mastery of key skills, knowledge, and attitudes. For many reasons, this model, which has long been in service in postgraduate medical education (PGME) training, is simply not valid any longer. In recognition of the need for change, countries around the world have started a dialogue about transitions to systems of competency-based education (CBE) or have already begun implementation. Examples of these include the Accreditation Council for Graduate Medical Education's (ACGME) Milestones Initiative[2], the Scottish Doctor project in the UK[3], and the Royal College of Physicians and Surgeons of Canada's Competence By Design initiative[4].

The drive to competency-based health professions education has been in response to a variety of pressures. These include the issue of work-hour restrictions, the advent of a much stronger focus on patient safety, enhanced educational approaches to programmatic assessment and curricular reform, and the aspiration to tailor the requirements at institutions involved in the training of health care professionals based on issues of social accountability. In the past 20 years, there has been a significant reduction in resident work hours principally in response to two overarching concerns. First, excessively long work hours are felt to be incompatible with optimizing resident learning and wellness, and second, although debated in the literature, there is the general belief that long work hours, and attendant resident fatigue and threats to overall physician wellness, are associated with higher incidences of medical error.[5-7] These issues have prompted a fundamental re-thinking of the traditional methods of training (i.e., time-based), and pose a question about whether new approaches can allow for flexibility in physician training. Time can be used more strategically and effectively while allowing residents to develop the competencies they require for independent practice while attaining work/life integration. This is something that is difficult to achieve under the current rigid training structures.

Within the current system, medical students are often assessed using Likert scale assessment tools, which rely on implicit standards that often vary between assessors and limit the amount of feedback that students receive.[8] To address this issue, in 2014, the Association of American Medical Colleges (AAMC) created "core entrustable professional activities (EPAs)."[9] These EPAs will help ensure that all medical students have the same competencies, and can be entrusted with the same tasks on their first days of residency training.

The current system of medical education in North America follows this pathway. Trainees enter medical school, where they receive a combination of basic human sciences teaching, an introduction to patient communication skills, variable clinical exposures, poorly defined faculty supervision, and often, inadequate clinical assessment. Also, despite their learning trajectories, there is no mechanism to alter the length of time required to begin PGME. Upon entry to residency, postgraduate medical trainees progress through a pre-determined clinical rotation schedule throughout their residency programs and are often provided with limited and/or sub-optimal feedback, inadequate faculty supervision, and in the worst circumstances, cursory summative assessments of their performance. Luckily though, most residents do progress satisfactorily along, despite not having ample and explicit evidence of competency attainment or mastery of skills in defined areas of their specialty.

In the current system, the status quo is the following: if a trainee hasn't created a red flag, then competency is assumed based on time spent on task. Unfortunately, this type of system structure creates a "failure to fail" culture,[10] which too often can occur, as noted in the AAMC's *Core Entrustable Professional Activities for Entering Residency – Curriculum Developers' Guide*. As a result of this culture, two problems emerge. The first is that a weak resident will progress through the training system much further than they should before they are identified. This makes remediation more difficult for multiple reasons: long delays, impacts on patient safety, and trainee resistance to support. Also, what may have been a simple fix had the trainee's difficulties been caught earlier, can become a deep-rooted trainee weakness that the current rigid time-based, rotation-specific system can't adequately address. The second problem that emerges is for residents who are excelling on trajectories above that of their peer group. For residents who are clearly progressing at a faster pace, the system does not allow for accelerated individualized pathways with further mastery of skills and/or earlier certification.

A 60-YEAR MOVEMENT TAKING MEDICINE BY STORM

Competency-based education (CBE) has been part of the educational landscape of higher education since it was first "introduced in America towards the end of the 1960s in reaction to concerns that students [were] not [being] taught the skills they require in life after school."[11] CBE has its roots in behaviorist/mastery learning theories of the 1960s and 70s, which suggested that most students have the ability to master a task or a skill given sufficient time and the appropriate methods and materials. In the 1970s, vocational programs targeting adult learners returning to college incorporated aspects of CBE by linking "educational progress to student performance rather than seat time by emphasizing learning outcomes (which were typically embedded in the curriculum) and the assessment of those outcomes."[12] Kate Ford has suggested that "until recently, CBE programs were primarily a niche offering targeting the adult learning segment of the higher education market space" but that "online learning, advances in learning analytics and adaptive learning technology, and the operationalization of direct assessment models to entire college degree programs"[13] have shifted CBE towards its current focus and applicability to all learners. These foci shifted CBE to a more constructivist approach where learners build knowledge or competencies.

Various industries have taken advantage of the flexibility and learner-centered focus provided by CBE as their professionals transition into new positions, or to enhance existing continuing educational development opportunities within companies. An early example of CBE was within the American military, where CBE enables military personnel to demonstrate their competencies in a way that is recognizable in the civilian community.[14] CBE also allows military veterans to reduce the time that they spend bridging the gap between their military experience and the credentials they need for their desired civilian careers, thereby ensuring that professionals with valuable skill sets spend less time in the classroom and more time putting those skills to use in the community.

The military's experiences with CBE spread to other areas as well, including the aviation industry.[15] As with medical education, aviation has traditionally operated on a time-based training model, with set amounts of flying time required for licensure. In the past decade, aviation training has become fully competency-based, which means that "industry newcomers experience training programs that are generally shorter and less expensive than their predecessors."[16] As there is expected to be increased air travel in the coming decades, the aviation industry faces a major shortage of pilots as well as mechanics and air traffic controllers. CBE training provides a way to accelerate the training process while maintaining high-quality training standards that are transparent and socially accountable.

As an educational framework, CBE is well-suited for lifelong learning and can help learners easily identify gaps in their existing knowledge. The outcomes-based, learner-centered approach of CBE has, since the last decade of the 20th century, begun to transform the health sciences pedagogical landscape. In the UK, this shift began in UGME with the Scottish Doctor's project, which began the process of developing outcomes in medical education as a response to the publication of

Tomorrow's Doctors[17] by the UK General Medical Council (GMC) in 1993. In Europe, The Turing Project is "funded by the European Commission to develop learning outcomes/competences for degree programmes" including medicine, "and to promote harmonisation in the higher education sector."[18]

In the United States, competency-based medical education has been largely focused on residency training since the ACGME launched the Milestones project in 1999, with the development of six general competencies endorsed by ACGME and the American Board of Medical Specialties (ABMS).[19] Also in 1999, the AAMC's Medical School Objectives Project (MSOP) produced a report advocating for competency-based education.[20] More recently, the Consortium of Accelerated Medical Pathway Programs (CAMPP), based out of New York University and supported by a Macy Foundation educational grant, is underway with the creation of novel accelerated paths that streamline UGME with entry into PGME at 12 separate medical schools.[21]

Within Canada, there has been a significant progression towards competency-based medical training as well. During the early 1990s, "Fellows of the Royal College, with support from the charitable institution, Associated Medical Services, leveraged the important work of the Educating Future Physicians for Ontario project to develop a competency framework for specialist physicians."[4] This resulted in the CanMEDS Framework, which articulated "the seven roles of the physician." Of note, these seven roles were also adopted by medical education jurisdictions in Australia, Denmark, the Netherlands, New Zealand, and the United Kingdom, as they redesigned their medical education curriculum.[22] The Royal College of Physicians & Surgeons of Canada launched the updated CanMEDS national framework at the International Conference on Residency Education (ICRE) in 2015, and the commencement of an ambitious national initiative, the Competence By Design (CBD) Project, that will see all postgraduate training programs becoming competency-based over the next five years. Examining how UGME will become streamlined with PGME within Canada, the Association of Faculties of Medicine in Canada (AFMC) have embarked on developing pan-Canadian EPAs for all medical school graduates as they embark upon their residency training.[23]

The new system of competency-based medical education will provide trainees with a mandate of regular assessment of competencies in a developmental progression, and will limit promotion unless specific competencies have been achieved. To provide support for trainees in this envisioned new system, there will be a comprehensive electronic assessment portfolio, individualized faculty mentors/advisors for each trainee, and a new competency committee framework that will explicitly examine each trainee's assessment portfolio, making promotion recommendations at regular intervals. As a result, each trainee will have a comprehensive, individualized, and flexible training plan that is learner-centered and evidence-based. To maintain the social contract health care institutions have with society, the demand for a higher threshold of demonstrated competency for independent medical practice is a must—something that is currently lacking in a world of rapidly changing health care systems. Moving forward, there must be improved explicit evidence for all trainees that documents their path to becoming a fully certified independent medical practitioner within their chosen specialty.

Not to be ignored in efforts to optimize trainee achievement of competency is the fundamental tension in the current system of graduate medical education of the service roles and responsibilities of residents in training. Are residents employees of the hospital who are primarily service providers, or are they work-based adult learners, who are principally there to attain professional competencies? While it has long been recognized that they are both, or more accurately, a hybrid between student and employee, the clinical imperative in most health care delivery settings has tended to create an imbalance towards service compared with education. Further separating the two, education was often delivered in a didactic, half-day, lecture-based format not based on adult learning principles. To this end, rather than looking at health care trainees as hospital service providers who happen to learn while they are in training, a shift in focus is needed to change the philosophy.

In a CBE system, learners are graduate medical education trainees who also provide hospital service as a fundamental work-based component of their educational program, wherein education and clinical work are integrated rather than separated. This is very different from the current model, and changing this view does not come without necessary revisions to the funding framework, to the provision of hospital-based patient care, and to the stated educational goals of health care institutions. Integration of these foundational elements is essential and it must be argued that service and education are not mutually exclusive.

FROM CONCEPT TO REALITY

A Systems Approach to Change Management

Undertaking a transition to a CBE curriculum can be a daunting task, and there are many ways to approach it. Institutions like Western Governors University were developed to be completely competency-based, with a mission that includes affordability for students and responsiveness to employers.[24] Other institutions implementing CBE programs, however, are doing so within current semester-based frameworks, but are focusing on outcomes based-learning and increasing the effectiveness and frequency of assessments. In thinking about optimal methods for transforming medical education programs, such as residency programs, to CBE, there have been several models contemplated. These include models that take a program-by-program approach; models that take an approach across a specific specialty; and a model that takes an approach across an entire learning institution, such as a university of academic health science center. The authors argue that a systems-wide approach for transforming postgraduate medical residency specialties, such as currently implemented at Queen's University, Canada, is optimal. By taking a holistic approach to innovations in health education, leaders and administrators within medical education can ensure that resources are allocated equally across programs, and perhaps more importantly, that faculty development and training programs can create equal educational experiences and expectations for residents across a school of medicine.

There are fundamental operational components to the implementation of CBE within health care institutions, regardless of the total number of specialty programs. First and foremost, time must not be used as the most important building block of a training program. Moving forward, it must be seen as an important resource, but only in combination with the optimization of teaching and learning environments, a comprehensive programmatic assessment strategy, and critical appraisal of what's most needed to attain a specialty's requisite competencies. Medical education leaders must ask themselves three key questions:

- Has there been critical reform of the curricular approach (rotations, required training experiences, elective time)?

- Has there been critical reform of the approach to assessment (multi-source feedback, developmental framework, timing of assessments, and use of electronic platforms)?

- Have EPAs been designed in a stage-wise progressive manner to represent the requisite competencies required for independent practice within a given specialty?

Without a thorough examination in these three domains, it cannot be said that CBE has been implemented.

CBE implementation also requires a comprehensive support structure. This includes strategic approaches to project leadership, faculty development, resident trainee engagement, academic scholarship, program evaluation, information technology systems, and a diverse and continuous approach to communications with all stakeholders. These foundational pillars are essential to the planning, implementation, and sustainability of the CBE change management process, and without them in place prior to implementation, the introduction of CBE to graduate medical education will not likely succeed.

An important aspect of CBE change management, too often forgotten or not fully grasped by change leaders, is that multiple groups of stakeholders need to be continually engaged and encouraged to take on leadership roles to get the work done. The impact of stakeholder engagement within CBE is far-reaching, and includes "the decanal leadership, hospital-based educational leadership, a CBE leadership team, program directors, CBE program leads, resident trainees in both the new and existing systems, program administrative assistants, department heads and division chairs, information technology staff, faculty development and continuing professional development leaders, undergraduate medical education leaders, and administrators and staff at affiliated teaching hospitals, including regional providers and hospitals. At the center of the stakeholders at our institution are the patients and their families."[25] The need for stakeholder communication also extends to regional/state-wide and national bodies to ensure consistent quality of care across geographic areas.

At the heart of stakeholder engagement is a belief in a shared purpose that unites the hearts and minds of communities of educators and care providers who can lead by example as they seek to modify the current culture of medical education.

The transition of health sciences education to CBE is an opportunity to build relationships and gather feedback that can continue to improve the quality of health education.

Critical to the national change process is engagement of government and other funders to help moderate the costs associated with increased training flexibility. As trainees move through their training on different trajectories, funding from grants and fellowships will need to be able to be applied with more flexibility.[26] At present, there is no buffer to a system that is overly rigid and inflexible. With varying times to completion possible with CBE, and the blurring of the margins for achieving additional complementary or subspecialty competencies, it will be imperative that governments provide funding to support lateral movement through short work-study programs. Large investments of government funds are not what will be needed to facilitate CBE training, but rather existing funding needs to be made more flexible and dynamic through pots of funding that can be allocated at the discretion of university health networks.

As change occurs, medical training programs and departments will need to test proof-of-concept experiences in the hospital care environments (operating room [OR], emergency department [ED], intensive care unit [ICU], patient wards, clinics, etc.), university learning environments (electronic learning libraries, simulation and reanimation labs, small group tutorial spaces, and large group auditorium classrooms), and within the community (offices, multi-disciplinary health centers) so that new and novel approaches to education can be shared across the health sciences training spectrum. No longer can inflexible, slow-to-adapt, time-proven traditions of medical teaching be honored as the gold standards of learning; newer, dynamic, adaptive, and creative solutions to teaching and learning are required for competency-based medical education to deliver on its promise of individualized learning for each trainee.

Interprofessional and Multi-Disciplinary Competencies

Interprofessional and multi-disciplinary competencies will be far more important as health sciences trainees will be working in more integrated team environments. The increasing complexity of medical care, the need for multiple team members with differing professional competencies to work together, and the imperative of a renewed patient- and family-centered care focus demands a change in competency training. Multi-disciplinary team approaches to care are the new reality for health care providers. Patient- and family-centered care demands that health care practitioners not only include patients and families in decision-making processes, but also that all members of a treatment team be included and informed of all treatment decisions. With increased specialization across the health care fields, it is more important than ever that health professionals develop competencies related to their roles as collaborators so that patients receive optimal continuity of care during treatment.

In the new realm of CBE, the integration of interprofessional and multi-disciplinary teams need not be conceived as requiring large structural changes to the current training system. Arguably, the building blocks are already there in the service provision of providing high-quality, team-based clinical care to patients and their families. Instead, what is needed is better inclusion of team members into the required training experiences and programmatic assessment process. The silo approach of physicians supervising and assessing physicians almost exclusively should end. For trainees to achieve many foundational, core, and junior attending level competencies, the interprofessional and multi-disciplinary team dynamic and synergistic components cannot be separated out, whether it be in the ED, OR, ICU, ward, or clinic environment. In a CBE model of training, all team members must be engaged in all aspects of the training experiences, supervision, and assessment processes, where appropriate, to capture the holistic realities and complexities of patient- and family-centered care, which is at the core of all service delivery.

New Technologies

As we move into the next 50 years of medical education, the technology that is available is changing the role of health care professionals and the competencies they will be required to master. In anesthesiology, for example, new "perioperative information management systems are used to display and store physiological monitoring data, drug administration data, details of procedures performed by anesthesia providers, patient demographic data, and other data obtained during anesthetic care."[27] With technology being able to manage aspects of the medical expert competencies for anesthesiologists, the other roles, including collaborator, health advocate, and scholar will expand. We need to prepare learners who will undoubtedly have to adapt to massive technologically driven changes that will fundamentally alter the current nature of their specialty work.

Researchers at the Universitat Politècnica de Catalunya are currently engaged in developing sensors that can be used to monitor heart rates and respiratory rates of patients who are elderly or disabled and living at home. These sensors can be hidden in furniture to be as minimally invasive to the patient as possible, and will allow them to continue safely living in their own homes.

Fitbit, the popular lifestyle gadget that allows users to track heart rate, daily steps, exercise, and calories, could find a new use as a medical diagnostic tool. A research team at Stanford University, led by Professor Michael Snyder, has discovered that the device may be able to detect when people are starting to get sick by looking at skin temperature and heart rate.[28] In the future, this kind of physiological monitoring may allow patients to use Fitbit and smartphone technology from home to upload their vitals, such as blood work and scans, to a care team. Unusual vitals would trigger an alert that would allow the monitoring team to provide appropriate care and also possibly deliver a wide array of home-based micro-medication doses similar to how diabetics today use subcutaneous insulin pumps.

Medical robots are increasingly being found in hospitals, operating rooms, and even in patient's homes. Magnetic Microbots can remove plaque from a patient's arteries or assist with ocular conditions and disease screenings. Service robots will move through hospital corridors making deliveries, and according to the Wall Street Journal, they are "self-aware, intelligent, and able to navigate changing environments, even chaotic hospital settings."[29] As the automation of highly skilled jobs increases, there may be concerns about technology completely overtaking jobs now held by human beings; a special report to The Economist, however, suggests that technology may end up creating more jobs than it destroys. David Autor, economist at the Massachusetts Institute of Technology, claims that "automating a particular task so that it can be done more quickly or cheaply, increases the demand for human workers to do the other tasks around it that have not been automated."[30] For example, radiologists who cannot compete with a computer's ability to diagnose abnormalities, might then transition from the task of reading and interpreting images to spending more time engaged directly with patients. This, quite possibly, could lead in the long term to fewer radiologists entering practice.

Similarly, new artificially intelligent supercomputers such as IBM Watson will be able to instantly search medical databases for literature that is relevant to the data entered by a physician. This will decrease the probability of missed diagnoses and eliminate physician bias. Since physicians will not have to spend as much time searching for the information they need, they will be able to increase the time that they spend with patients, thereby increasing the quality of the information they can feed into Watson.[31]

Further, interactive 3D holograms can assist with diagnoses, and with pre-surgical planning, letting physicians see a true 3D model of what they can expect when they get into the operating room, something that in the past we could only imagine from science fiction literature. Additionally, patients may find these kinds of models easier to understand than 2D medical images, which will improve a patient's understanding of procedures and treatment options in a more comprehensive way.[32] In fact, "holographic interferometric techniques have been widely applied with success for the study of different parts of the human body, including cornea, tooth mobility, tympanic membrane, basilar membrane, cochlea, temporal bone, incudo-mallar joint, chest, skull, and bones."[33] With this kind of technology available now, it seems likely that, in the next 50 years, these images will benefit health care professionals serving remote populations. 3D holographic images could be sent from remote areas to larger urban centers for consultation, and applications that allow users to share their computer screens could be used to demonstrate surgical procedures on the hologram to teach less specialized doctors to perform lifesaving procedures.

For medical students and residents entering training today, familiarity and competency with these new technologies will be necessary for their future practices. It may not be long before holographic imagery is used in high-fidelity simulation training, reducing the number of human volunteers and computerized mannequins that are needed, while also optimizing the fidelity of the training environment, which is greatly needed. As technology continues to evolve, simulation training will be required not only for students and graduate residents, but also for all independent healthcare practitioners as part of their continuing professional development. In fact, in a CBE world, the competencies themselves will aid the transitions to new technologies and practices.

Curriculum Renewal and Innovation

With the transition to CBE, medical education at both the undergraduate and graduate levels will require significant curricular reform (clinical rotations, teaching and learning environments, required training experiences, elective experiences, and more) both from within traditional training programs, immediately following medical school, and for post-residency competency training initiatives for independent practitioners. As technology continues to develop at a rapid pace, lifelong learning will become increasingly important to physicians as they will need to be continuously changing and adapting to new roles. Sebastian Thrun, a professor at Stanford, suggests that "people will have to continuously learn new skills to stay current," which is one of the reasons Thrun's firm focuses on "nano-degrees… which can be completed in a few months, alongside a job."[34] Online courses can provide increased access to learning opportunities, but truly the vision of the future should be to open up diverse opportunities for re-entry to training and work/study programs. Currently, these opportunities are quite limited and this fundamentally needs to change.

How can society expect specialists to develop new competencies across multiple physician roles (see Table 1 for examples of competencies) without being immersed in the clinical environment of care delivery? Is it possible for small-group classroom sessions, multi-day conference courses, or online modules to effectively provide the required training experiences to attain new EPAs, and/or other specialized competencies, if they are offered away from the patient care areas where the integration of multiple physician roles truly takes place? CBE medical training demands the possibility of multiple streams of short-, medium-, and longer-term training programs that are offered in the clinical context, supplemented by simulation experiences, and that limit exposure to non-patient contact learning. It must also not be limited to discrete or finite periods of time immediately following medical school. Smith, Stockley, Flynn, and McDiarmid[35] argue that health care practitioners trained in CBE will require sustainable professional activities that "reflect the continuing professional development process required to sustain a competent practicing physician." These "Sustainable Professional Activities will require different skills for physicians, including the ability to continuously incorporate new evidence, interrogate their practice, seek new knowledge, refine and revise their practice." At the same time as different skills are needed, some professional activities will no longer be needed for a practicing physician. A national portfolio system will make it easier for health care practitioners to identify competencies they need to update or maintain.

Table 1 - Sample Competencies Frameworks in Medical Education

CANADA (RCPSC)	UNITED STATES (ACGME)	SCOTLAND	AUSTRALIA (AMA)
Medical Educator	Patient Care and Procedural Skills	Delivering the Service	Patient-Doctor Trust Relationship
Scholar	Medical Knowledge	Demonstrating Personal Qualities	Diagnosis & Prognosis
Communicator	Practice-Based Learning and Improvement	Working with Others	Complex Decision Making
Health Advocate	Systems-based Practice	Managing Services	Multi-Disciplinary Approach
Professional	Professionalism	Improving Services	Professionalism
Leader	Interpersonal Skills and Communication	Setting Direction	Leadership in Health Services & Community
Collaborator			Training the Next generation
			Medical Education as Lifelong Learning

As part of an ongoing process of educational development, assessment for both students and faculty will move to online portfolio management systems. Assessments and encounters can be entered to provide real-time, two-way feedback as preceptors and faculty can provide assessments to trainees, while trainees can provide feedback on the usefulness of faculty assessments. Aggregate data compiled from the portfolios can be used to compare students within programs and across institutions, and can be used to develop ongoing program evaluation for continual improvement of training programs—and possibly for program accreditation. A national portfolio system can be used across the career of a health care practitioner to help them identify gaps in competencies, and to ensure maintenance of competencies already attained. Additionally, it is easy to envision a new model of continuing professional development that offers mentorship opportunities for newly certified independent practitioners, and for all physicians who seek guidance on their career trajectories over many years. With electronic portfolios, normative data curves, well-defined competencies across all specialty areas, and a strategy to ongoing brief but individualized mentorship, CBE will continue well beyond medical school and residency training to include all practicing physicians for the duration of their careers.

The current organization of medical education in most jurisdictions is not congruent with modern-day thinking about competency progression. The silos are rigid. In North America, for the most part, the pathway to becoming a practicing physician includes very discrete, non-integrated stages including an undergraduate first-entry degree, UGME, postgraduate residency training, fellowship training, and often the attainment of a graduate degree, either before medical school or during or after residency.

We can envision a less discrete continuum that would see the possible merging of a first-entry degree with UGME, the transition to specialty training happening at some point in medical school, and a more flexible approach to residency training that might well incorporate early subspecialization or academic training. Indeed, there are several examples of these kinds of initiatives happening currently. They are, however, all in a pilot phase, and currently national standards, for the most part, stultify creativity in a new design of training. Additionally, we envision the creation of new nano-programs, which can supplement the existing competencies of a health care practitioner by permitting someone to engage in national work/study programs without having to update provincial or state licenses.

In North America, postgraduate medical training takes place within hospitals or clinics under the supervision of more experienced physicians. This apprenticeship model is a useful one, but as we transition to a CBE framework for training, we need to recognize that we are asking faculty to teach in a system that is new and unfamiliar, since they were not trained this way. Given the relative unfamiliarity of practicing clinicians with many of the pedagogical necessities of CBE, it will be imperative for universities to play a fundamental role in partnering with hospitals and other care environments for the transfer of knowledge and expertise, especially in competency assessment.

THE FUTURE IS NOW

Over the past decade, health care professionals internationally have recognized that the traditional way of educating health care practitioners is in need of change. The fundamental structure of medical education has not changed in nearly a century and much has changed since then. The need to reduce training times and the prioritization of physician wellness, combined with rapidly changing technological innovations, have made apparent the cracks in the current education model, and have highlighted the need for significant changes in health education.

With its flexibility and learner-centered focus, CBE provides a unique opportunity to transform health sciences education and training. With its focus on accruing specific competencies rather than following specific timelines, CBE can create opportunities for physicians to become more well-rounded and versatile health care professionals. Programs in a CBE model will graduate physicians with confidence that the specific competencies needed for the practice of a specialty have been acquired. In an era of increased accountability, a CBE model will provide firm evidence of graduating practitioners skilled in a suite of EPAs within a framework of agreed-to competencies. It also will allow physicians to better serve their patients and communities by enabling them to acquire the novel sets of competencies that are necessary to provide quality care in their unique local contexts.

Physicians will become empowered to adapt their skill sets according to these local contexts, thus increasing their sense of work satisfaction while demonstrating ongoing career development. Lastly, physicians will be able to establish greater work-life integration by having the flexibility to attend to their personal and professional needs or interests, without compromising their competence or confidence to provide quality patient care. Taken together, a fully integrated competency-based medical education approach results in better health for physicians and better and safer care for their patients.

While some of what we've envisioned in this paper may take decades to achieve, we need to start laying the groundwork now to make this future a reality. These changes start at the institutional level by engaging stakeholders and having them invest in CBE. As part of this stakeholder engagement, we also need to break down the silos between programs and specialties, and start thinking about multi-disciplinary approaches to health care that can engage people across these boundaries. At the same time, we need to start advocating for increased flexibility and discretionary power in how government funds are allocated and used for training. As health sciences education transitions to CBE, we need to focus on collaboration locally, nationally, and internationally. We have an opportunity to move beyond institutional protectionism, and to train the global doctors of tomorrow.

Years later at Jane's 20th medical school reunion, she was amazed that many of her classmates had become full-time educators, some administrators, and others had developed competencies in many different secondary specialties and other health care professions, regardless of what discipline they started in. It seemed that the lines of separation between the traditional health care professions had become quite blurred and crossover between disciplines was much less rigid than in the previous generation.

With a focus on accruing specific competencies rather than time spent in specialty areas, competency-based education successfully created the opportunity for physicians to become much more versatile health care professionals. This versatility proved to be more patient-centered and also physician-friendly compared with previous training models. It allowed physicians to better serve their patients and communities through acquiring novel sets of competencies that were necessary to provide quality care in their local contexts. Physicians also felt empowered to adapt their skill sets according to these local contexts, thus increasing their sense of work satisfaction. Lastly, physicians were able to establish a greater work-life integration by having the flexibility to attend to their personal and professional needs or interests, without compromising their competence or confidence to provide quality patient care. Taken together, a fully integrated competency-based medical education approach resulted in greater happiness and health for both physicians and their patients.

ACKNOWLEDGEMENTS

The authors thank Dr. Debra Klamen (Southern Illinois University School of Medicine) and Dr. George Mejicano (Oregon Health & Science University) for their thorough reviews of earlier versions of this paper.

REFERENCES

1. Snell LS, Frank JR. Competencies, the tea bag model, and the end of time. *Med Teach.* 2010;32(8):629–630.

2. Milestones [Internet]. [cited 2017 Feb 7]. Available from: http://www.acgme.org/What-We-Do/Accreditation/Milestones/Overview

3. The Scottish Doctor [Internet]. [cited 2017 Feb 24]. Available from: http://www.scottishdoctor.org/

4. The Royal College of Physicians and Surgeons of Canada: Competence by Design [Internet]. [cited 2017 Feb 24]. Available from: http://www.royalcollege.ca/rcsite/competence-design-e

5. West CP, Huschka MM, Novotny PJ, et al. Association of perceived medical errors with resident distress and empathy: A prospective longitudinal study. *JAMA* 2006;296(9):1071–1078.

6. West CP, Tan AD, Habermann TM, Sloan JA, Shanafelt TD. Association of resident fatigue and distress with perceived medical errors. *JAMA* 2009; 302(12):1294–1300.

7. Williams ES, Manwell LB, Konrad TR, Linzer M. The relationship of organizational culture, stress, satisfaction and burnout with physician-reported error and suboptimal patient care: Results from the MEMO Study. *Health Care Manage Rev.* 2007;32(3):203–212.

8. Toprak A, Luhanga U, Jones S, Winthrop, A, & McEwen, L. Validation of a novel intraoperative assessment tool: The Surgical Procedure Feedback Rubric. *Am J Surg.* 2016;211(2):369–376. https://doi.org/10.1016/j.amjsurg.2015.08.032

9. Association of American Medical Schools. Core Entrustable Professional Activities for Entering Residency – Curriculum Developers' Guide. 2014.

10. Dudek N. L., Marks, MB.; Regehr, G. V. Failure to fail: The perspectives of clinical supervisors. *Acad Med.* 2005 80:10:S84–S87.

11. Malan S. The "new paradigm" of outcomes-based education in perspective. *Tydskrif vir Gesinsekologie en Verbruikerswetenskappe.* 2000;28:22–28.

12. Nodine TR. How did we get here? A brief history of competency-based higher education in the United States. *J Competency-Based Educ.* 2016;1(1):5–11.

13. Ford K. Competency-Based Education: History, Opportunities, and Challenges. UMUC Center for Innovation in Learning and Student Success (CILSS); 2014.

14. Seal M. How CBE Helps Bridge the Gap Between Military Experience and Civilian Credentials [Internet]. Ellucian | The leader in higher education technology. 2016 [cited 2017 Feb 9]. Available from: http://www.ellucian.com/Blog/How-CBE-helps-bridge-the-gap-between-military-experience-and-civilian-credentials/

15. Jackson CR, Gibbon KP. Training tomorrow's surgeons using inter alia lessons from aviation. *J Roy Soc Med*. 2006;99:554–558.

16. Mavin APT, Hodge DS, Kearns DSK. Competency-Based Education in Aviation: Exploring Alternate Training Pathways. Ashgate Publishing, Ltd.; 2016. 240 p.

17. General Medical Council. Tomorrow's Doctors: Outcomes and Standards for Undergraduate Medical Education [Internet]. 2009 [cited 2017 Feb 7]. Available from: http://www.gmc-uk.org/Tomorrow_s_Doctors_1214.pdf_48905759.pdf

18. Cumming A, Cumming A, Ross M. The Tuning Project for Medicine–Learning outcomes for undergraduate medical education in Europe. *Med Teach*. 2007;29(7):636–641.

19. Holmboe E, Edgar L, Hamstra S. Milestones Guidebook.pdf [Internet]. 2016 [cited 2017 Feb 7]. Available from: http://www.acgme.org/Portals/0/MilestonesGuidebook.pdf

20. Morcke AM, Dornan T, Eika B. Outcome (competency) based education: An exploration of its origins, theoretical basis, and empirical evidence. *Adv Health Sci Educ Theory Pract*. 2013;18:851–863.

21. Consortium of Medical Schools with Accelerated Pathway Programs [Internet]. [cited 2017 Feb 26]. Available from: http://macyfoundation.org/grantees/profile/consortium-of-medical-schools-with-accelerated-pathway-programs

22. Scheele F, Teunissen P, Van Luijk S, et al. Introducing competency-based postgraduate medical education in the Netherlands. *Med Teach*. 2008;30:248–253.

23. Association of Faculties of Medicine of Canada. AFMC Entrustable Professional Activities for the Transition from Medical School to Residency. Available: https://afmc.ca/sites/default/files/documents/AFMC_Entrustable_Professional_Activities_EN_0.pdf

24. What is CBE? [Internet]. CBEinfo.org. [cited 2017 Feb 26]. Available from: http://www.cbeinfo.org/what-is-cbe.html

25. Dagnone D, Walker R, Flynn L, et al. Building capacity for cbme implementation at Queen's University. MedEdPublish [Internet]. 2017;6. Available from: http://www.mededpublish.org/manuscripts/808/v1

26. Bevan H, Fairman S. White Paper: The New Era of Thinking and Practice in Change and Transformation - A call to Action for Leaders of Health and Care [Internet]. *The Edge*. 2016 [cited 2017 Feb 26]. Available from: http://theedge. nhsiq.nhs.uk/white-paper-the-new-era-of-thinking-and-practice-in-change-and-transformation-a-call-to-action-for-leaders-of-health-and-care/

27. Wanderer JP, Ehrenfeld JM. Clinical Decision Support for Perioperative Information Management Systems. *Semin Cardiothorac Vasc Anesth*. 2013;17(4):288–293.

28. Adams S. After the Fitbit, it's the "Sickbit" [Internet]. *Mail Online*. 2017 [cited 2017 Feb 8]. Available from: http://www.dailymail.co.uk/~/article-4167286/index.html

29. McNickle M. 10 Medical Robots That Could Change Healthcare [Internet]. *InformationWeek*. 2012 [cited 2017 Feb 8]. Available from: http://www. informationweek.com/healthcare/mobile-wireless/10-medical-robots-that-could-change-heal/240143983

30. Autor D. Automation and Anxiety [Internet]. *The Economist*. 2016 [cited 2017 Feb 8]. Available from: http://www.economist.com/news/special-report/21700758-will-smarter-machines-cause-mass-unemployment-automation-and-anxiety

31. Keim B. Paging Dr. Watson: Artificial Intelligence as a Prescription for Health Care [Internet]. *WIRED*. 2012 [cited 2017 Feb 8]. Available from: https://www.wired.com/2012/10/watson-for-medicine/

32. Handwerk B. Medical Holograms are Now Part of the Surgeon's Toolkit [Internet]. *Smithsonian*. 2015 [cited 2017 Feb 8]. Available from: http://www.smithsonianmag.com/science-nature/medical-holograms-are-now-part-surgeons-toolkit-180954791/

33. Mehta P. Medical Applications of Holography [Internet]. INTEGRAF. 2005 [cited 2017 Feb 8]. Available from: http://www.integraf.com/resources/articles/a-medical-applications-of-holography

34. Autor D. Re-educating Rita [Internet]. The Economist. 2016 [cited 2017 Feb 8]. Available from: http://www.economist.com/news/special-report/21700760-artificial-intelligence-will-have-implications-policymakers-education-welfare-and

35. Smith K, Stockley D, Flynn L, McDiarmid L. Sustainable Professional Activities. *Med Teach*. 2016 Aug 2;38(8):859.

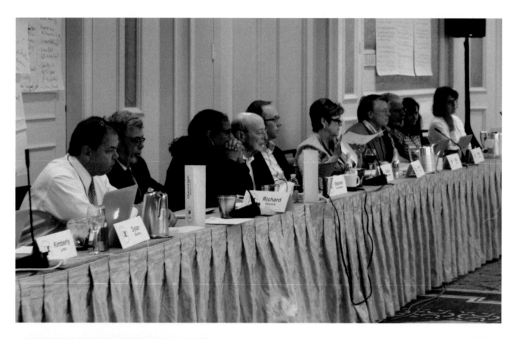

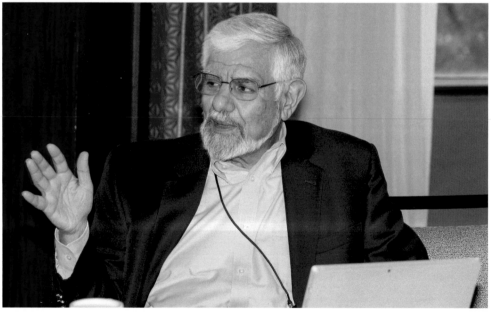

THE UNIVERSITY OF WISCONSIN-MILWAUKEE

FLEXIBLE OPTION FOR BSN COMPLETION

Case Study

Kim Litwack, PhD, RN, FAAN
Dean, UWM College of Nursing and

Aaron M. Brower, PhD
Provost and Vice Chancellor, UW-Extension

In 2014, the University of Wisconsin-Milwaukee (UWM) launched the UW Flexible (Flex) Option for BSN Completion. The purpose of this paper is to examine the history of our decision to consider and launch the Flex Option as a competency-based delivery approach to RN-BSN completion, including factors that contributed to its success, discussion of obstacles, and identification of continued challenges that have yet to be resolved.

RN-BSN COMPLETION: RATIONALE

Among its recommendations, the *Future of Nursing* report by the Institute of Medicine (IOM) recommends that 80% of registered nurses have a Bachelor of Science in Nursing (BSN) degree by the year 2020.[1] This goal was rooted in research indicating that patients receive better care in hospitals where the majority of nurses have higher-level academic degrees. Nurse researchers found that every 10 percent increase in the proportion of BSN nurses on the hospital staff was associated with a four percent decrease in the risk for death.[2] Currently, only 55% of nurses hold degrees at the baccalaureate level and above.[3]

The American Nurses Credentialing Center (ANCC), an affiliate of the American Nurses Association, gives the prestigious Magnet status to hospitals that satisfy criteria that measure the strength and quality of their nursing services. The program goals of Magnet are to 1) recognize excellence in the delivery of nursing services to patients; 2) promote quality in a milieu that supports professional clinical practice, and 3) provide a mechanism for disseminating best practices in nursing services.[4] In Magnet hospitals, approximately 50% of all nurses associated with direct care have a BSN.

At this time, the ANCC does not specify degree requirements for direct-care providers, nor does it specify the percentage of nurses who must hold a BSN degree, but it does require that 100% of the organization's nurse managers have a BSN or graduate degree. Some hospitals have mirrored the IOM goal of 80% of nurses with BSNs, anticipating the requirement that, by 2020, Magnet hospitals will need to ensure 80% of its nurses hold a BSN degree. That said, the clear trend is toward employing baccalaureate-prepared nurses in the clinical environments of Magnet hospitals, and hospitals are preferentially hiring BSN graduates over associate degree (ADN) graduates or are hiring ADN graduates with the mandated expectation that these nurses commit to returning to school. Initiatives like "BSN in 3" or "BSN in 5" (as in three or five years) are driving hiring expectations.[5]

BARRIERS TO RN TO BSN COMPLETION

According to a study published in the *Journal of Nursing Administration*, the four main barriers to pursuing a BSN are financial constraints, competing priorities, past academic experience, and lack of academic support.[6] Financial constraints include the cost of the academic program, as well as the potential need to reduce hours of work to attend classes. Competing priorities include work hours and rotating shifts, school hours, family commitment hours, and volunteer hours. Past academic experience includes academic performance in previous degree programs as well as the experience of attending school in the past. Inadequate access to tutoring, writing assistance, and test-taking strategies are examples of lack of academic support.

Other barriers include lack of employer support (no adjustment in work hours; schedule demands; no tuition support or acknowledgement in salary after degree completion) and insecurity about the ability to be successful.[7] Given the push toward BSN as the preferred degree, it is important that hospital partners and educational facilities work together to identify strategies to support completion by not only addressing barriers, but also supporting motivators for completion. The same authors who identified the barriers also identified motivators to BSN completion, including length of program, financial compensation or tuition reimbursement, and encouragement from family members.[6]

OUR HISTORY IN BSN COMPLETION

The UWM College of Nursing (CON) has a long history of supporting BSN completion by removing and addressing barriers to finishing the BSN degree. We now offer BSN completion in three modes: BSN@Home, BSN@Work, and the UW Flexible (Flex) Option.

The **BSN@Home** is an online program offered in partnership with five other University of Wisconsin (UW) campuses that also offer nursing programs. This partnership provides a shared online curriculum of upper-level nursing courses along with a home campus mode to fulfill other requirements for the Bachelor of Science degree. By sharing the delivery of the courses, each campus benefits from the others' faculty expertise and a shared workload. Students enrolled at UWM receive their advising, financial aid, and other student support services through UWM. Courses are offered during the fall, spring, and summer semesters. All the nursing courses can be taken online except for the final capstone seminar and practicum courses, taken in the final semester of the program. Offered in a hybrid format, this course requires students to attend four on-campus sessions in addition to online work and clinical practicum hours.

The flexibility of the online program allows students to balance work and family life while earning their bachelor's degree. The online program is asynchronous, allowing nurses to complete coursework on their own schedules; is offered at a lower online fee in lieu of tuition cost; and allows students to enroll at the start of any given semester.[8]

The **BSN@Work** option is a face-to-face delivery mode offering classes on-site at local area hospitals and technical colleges. When possible, nurses enroll as a cohort and progress together through courses. Now offered at three area hospitals, this program offering was recently changed to a seven-week course format, allowing students the ability to complete two courses per semester. In the past, when offered in a full semester mode, students typically took only one course per semester, delaying time to degree completion. The benefits of this mode of delivery are clear employer support and convenience, with courses offered at the workplace. The seven-week format allows a more rapid progression through the program.

BSN@Work has also been extended to a course offering in the face-to-face format at the local community college, in a unique collaboration with the community college considered the "work-site" for students. An elective UWM leadership course is co-taught by faculty from both the community college and UWM. The course meets a requirement for both the ADN degree as well as giving students a "jump-start" on BSN completion coursework. These students are tracked through a dedicated UWM advisor to facilitate degree progression and a smooth transfer into UWM.

COMPETENCY-BASED BSN COMPLETION: UW FLEXIBLE (FLEX) OPTION

In December 2013, the College of Nursing launched a third mode of delivery for BSN completion, the **UW Flexible (Flex) Option**. This is a self-paced, competency-based degree completion option that allows registered nurses to progress towards their BSN degree by demonstrating knowledge acquired through prior coursework, military training, on-the-job training, and other learning experiences. Students progress through the degree by successfully completing a series of competency assessments that demonstrate mastery of required knowledge and skills. No credit or grade will be given until all competency assessments within a given competency set have been completed and passed. This is NOT academic credit for life lived or previous nursing experience. The Flex Option allows students to receive credit only upon demonstration of clearly defined competencies required of BSN-prepared nurses. It is an innovative way to make BSN completion more accessible, convenient, and affordable for adult and non-traditional students.

All the routes for RN-BSN completion are grounded in the principles of adult learning. Adults prefer learning situations that are practical and problem-centered, promote their self-esteem, integrate new ideas with existing knowledge, show respect for individual learners, capitalize on their experience, and allow choice and self-direction.[9] Although a dated, but seminal reference, Malcolm Knowles observed that adult learners learn best when they understand *why* something is important; when they have the freedom to learn in their own way; when learning is experiential; when the time is right for them to learn, and when the process is positive and encouraging.[10] While all modes of RN-BSN delivery consider the principles of adult learning, only the Flex Option, utilizing competency-based education (CBE), embraces all five of Knowles' principles. The BSN@Home and the Flex Option allow students to learn when the time is right. The critical difference in the Flex Option is the freedom for students to learn their own way.

It might also be argued that the delivery modes will appeal to different types of students and their personal learning styles. Learning styles have been defined in numerous, often competing, ways. The BSN@Work face-to-face option may prove beneficial and more appealing to the student who prefers an engaged, social, interactive approach, requiring a time commitment and structure to learning. The BSN@Home online option may prove beneficial to a more self-directed student with competing time demands, who is comfortable with online engagement and the structure the online delivery system requires. The Flex Option appeals to the student who is self-directed, internally motivated, comfortable with limited but available engagement, and who is able to set their own schedule for learning as opposed to being boxed into a traditional academic schedule and calendar.

The faculty and staff who work with Flex students identified several characteristics of the students who were successful in that option. These students tended to be independent, self-directed critical thinkers with strong intrinsic motivation and attitude, who also had a support system, economic stability, a sense of ownership, time management skills, realistic expectations, determination, engagement in learning, and "grit."

DIFFERENT EDUCATIONAL MODALITY: SAME FACULTY AND EDUCATIONAL GOALS

The Flex Option is one of three delivery modes to the same endpoint: the BSN degree. Each delivery mode—online, face-to-face, and Flex—is grounded in the AACN baccalaureate essentials with identical program outcomes.[11] Each mode offers the same courses, uses the same objectives, and grants equivalent credits toward the baccalaureate degree. The delivery mode is the variable, with evaluation mechanisms within each delivery mode designed to support the specific approach. As an example, a face-to-face student may be able to deliver a presentation to classmates; an online student may upload a voice-over PowerPoint presentation, and a Flex Option student may provide the PowerPoint presentation without voice-over, but with notes to demonstrate competency within the course. It is reinforced to students that the curriculum is not changing, but instead, one additional delivery mode has been created for degree completion.

Currently there are seven required advanced nursing courses/competency sets (21 credits). A competency set is equivalent to a course in terms of objectives and credits. A set of three to four defined assessments for each course makes up a competency set. Satisfactory completion of the set results in the awarding of credits. In addition, students must complete a minimum of nine credits (three courses/competency sets) of advanced nursing electives (Table 1).

Table 1: Required and Elective Nursing Course

REQUIRED	ELECTIVE
Foundations of Professional Nursing Practice	Health Assessment
Leadership and Management	Global Health: Ethics and Human Rights
Research and Evidenced- Based Practice	Symptom Management for Chronic and Life-Limiting Illness
Community Health Nursing	Genetics and Genomics for Health Professionals
Information Management and Healthcare Technology	Mental Health Nursing Across the Care Continuum
Chronic Care Management	
Capstone/Practicum	

Students may enroll in one set or multiple sets at the beginning of every month, and have three months to complete the set. Tuition is priced for one set or for an "all-you-can-learn" model that allows students to register for as many sets as they feel they can complete in the three months. The three-month period of enrollment is referred to as a "subscription period."

UWM began enrolling students in the Flex Option program in early 2014. To date, over 1,000 unique students have enrolled in the Flex Option, completing 2,429 competency sets (courses). The first student to graduate using the Flex Option was able to complete her degree in 11 months, using her ADN degree credits as well as additional undergraduate credits and the 30 upper-division Flex nursing credits. Another is on track to finish in seven months. As of May 2017, 25 students have graduated from the Flex Option BSN degree program. The median completion rate for graduates from initial enrollment to graduation is 18 months; the mean is 16 months. As the program is relatively new and there is great variation in the number of transfer credits students bring to this option, these numbers are skewed and may change over time. Demographics of Flex students to date are consistent with those of our students in other BSN completion routes, in terms of gender, race, and age (Table 2).

Table 2: Flex Student Demographics

GENDER	88% female	12% male
RACE	92% Caucasian	8% Students of Color
AGE	Younger than age 25	7%
	25-30	27%
	31-35	23%
	36-40	17%
	41-45	11%
	46-50	8%
	50+	5%

The driving force behind the Flex Option was to provide registered nurses with an additional option for BSN completion, in consideration of factors identified by nurses that prevent their returning to school. This option is consistent with the need to be convenient, to minimize time constraints, and to be compatible with a registered nurse's often inconsistent work schedule. Because many registered nurses are non-traditional students with past college credits, who are working fulltime and who often have families, traditional educational approaches do not always meet their needs.

As the mode of delivery is asynchronous and self-directed, nurses progress at the speed they determine to be the best for them personally. Those who feel they need more time on a topic may take that time, while others who are ready to demonstrate mastery can do so. This is not learning by "seat time," but through demonstration of mastery. In addition, students may begin a competency set on the first day of every month, avoiding the need to wait until the start of a traditional semester. It is well-known that any delays in enrollment may result in a student not enrolling.[12]

The delivery mode of the Flex Option is less expensive than traditional online or face-to-face delivery options. A single, three-credit competency set costs $900, with students allowed three months to complete the set. For those who may be more motivated or have more time to commit, the Flex Option offers an "all-you-can-learn" option, also for three months, for $2,250. The "all-you-can-learn" option allows students to successfully master as many competency sets as they can within a three-month period. This is ideal for motivated learners who would like to earn their degrees more quickly. This cost can be contrasted with the online, three-credit course fee of $1,356 and a face-to-face course fee of $1,011.39. A face-to-face, on-campus, three-credit course tuition is $1,631.72 (January 2017). This is not a loss to the CON for tuition, as these students are new students who previously had not considered either the face-to-face or online options. In fact, it is our largest growth area and we are now marketing in additional states. This expansion will be done such that we ensure that revenue will cover the expenses of expansion, including maintaining our current commitment to individualized student success.

ESSENTIAL PROACTIVE AND WRAPAROUND SUPPORT: THE ACADEMIC SUCCESS COACH

It must be emphasized that students are not simply registering and then moving through the Flex Option without support. Through intrusive advising and regular, substantive interaction with set faculty and an academic success coach (ASC), the student is guided through competency set completion. Intrusive advising refers to purposeful, preemptive, proactive engagement with a student even before the student enrolls in the Flex Option and continuing at regular, defined intervals. The

ASC is more than a student advisor, thus the name "coach." The ASC provides a unique blend of academic advising, generalized tutoring, referral and administrative direction, and mentoring support throughout the duration of students' programs. ASCs help students understand their curricular paths and how best to succeed in a competency-based model. ASCs also connect students with the academic and administrative services they need as they progress through their academic programs. Set faculty engage with the student within three days of enrolling, and continue engaging regularly, with feedback on every assessment in a timely manner, as well as communication about set progress, expectations, and plans.

To offer the Flex Option, UWM works in partnership with, and with the support of, UW Extension. UW Extension works with all 26 UW campuses, providing, among other things, e-learning (online courses) for degree completion as well as three different online degrees. UW Extension also develops and administers collaborative degrees across all 26 UW campuses (online degrees that function similarly to the BSN@Home). Through this role, UW Extension has developed the administrative and "back office" capacity (instructional designers, instructional technologists, online recruiters and admissions personnel, bursar and financial aid counselors, and the student information system) to create and support Flex programs offered throughout the UW campuses for the UW Flex Option.[13] UW Flex Option programs are partnership programs: UW Extension provides administrative leadership and each UW campus provides academic leadership for their partnership program.

Currently, five degree programs and three certificates are offered through the UW Flex Option. In addition to the RN-to-BSN program highlighted in this case study, UW Flex offers a bachelors in diagnostic imaging, a bachelors in information technology, and a certificate in business and technical communications—all through UWM; a certificate in substance abuse disorders counseling through UW-Madison; an associate's degree in arts and sciences through the UW Colleges; a project management certificate through UW-Parkside; and a bachelors in business administration directly through UW-Extension.[14]

FACTORS THAT CONTRIBUTED TO THE SUCCESS

The launch and subsequent success of the Flex Option was not without deliberate attention to several factors. The CON is known for its innovative educational programming, including the launch of the first Doctor of Nursing Practice degree in the state system, the conversion of the undergraduate curriculum to a concept-based, competency model, the BSN@Home Consortial Program, and the launch of the nation's first online, asynchronous PhD program. In fact, it was the CON dean who volunteered to take on the challenge of developing the Flex Option and brought the initiative back to the faculty.

The UW system is grounded in shared governance, so any curricular change required the commitment and approval of the faculty. The faculty seized the opportunity and responded with an enthusiastic "yes" to working on making this idea a reality. Focusing on a post-licensure curriculum with fewer clinical requirements than those of pre-licensure programs was also important in selecting this learning mode. Our long history of BSN completion helped assure our clinical partners of our intent to succeed and our commitment to finding a third option for BSN completion. The leadership of not only the CON, but the university itself, including the chancellor and provost, supported the commitment to innovative change.

The faculty were committed to the success of the Flex Option. A dedicated faculty member took on leadership of the Flex Option, in addition to maintaining the BSN@Home and BSN@Work, in her role as director of BSN completion programs. Having a director who was already knowledgeable about the BSN completion curriculum was invaluable in keeping the process moving forward. She possessed a deep understanding of the BSN essentials[12] as well as every course offered to BSN completion students. In fact, the BSN@Home curriculum had been recently revised, so the curriculum was as current as it could be, reflecting the new essentials, which is the foundation of accreditation. This director was attentive, responsive, and very goal-directed. Her communication with stakeholders both internal to UWM, as well as external, including hospital partners, and UW-Extension kept this program on track and contributed to its success and our plans to expand.

Although the faculty had course objectives from the traditional online and face-to-face courses, faculty had to think differently, as they developed assessments that allowed the student to demonstrate competency mastery. Faculty first had to determine the essence of the competencies being learned in order then to build assessments that would allow students to demonstrate their mastery of those competencies. Faculty development workshops facilitated this work. Presentations were replaced with case studies. Those who typically used exams in their classes had to think about exam security and monitoring. Faculty were not teaching in the traditional sense, but needed to develop their competency sets in such a way as to guide learning and confirm mastery.

Competency-based assessment is a very different way of working with students. While faculty maintained independence over their competency sets, we discovered early on that consistency across the curriculum (i.e., curricular integrity) was the key to success. Each competency set used the same syllabus template. All faculty used the same template for loading their competency sets into our learning management system. All sets began with a PowerPoint orientation with notes. Each competency set had three to four learning assessments. Each assessment had a consistent learning path and an evaluation rubric. Regardless of the set being completed, students were quick to see that each set looked similar, with the same functional template, same level of detail of instructions, clear requirements for completion, and grading rubrics for each assessment. Team meetings kept faculty consistent, and each new faculty member to join the Flex team was orientated to the Flex philosophy, learning strategies, and assessment models.

There were a number of supports in place to assist faculty and the success of the program. Other individuals from UWM that contributed to the successful launch included the registrar, who facilitated posting of grades on a non-academic calendar and transcript designations; financial aid representatives, as the Flex Option posed unique challenges for financial aid; and the CON's assistant dean for business affairs who helped with financial modeling. Instructional designers helped ensure consistency of the electronic platform.

The launch required not only the commitment of individuals within UWM, but also the support of the UW Extension on behalf of the UW system. As stated, Flex Option programs are partnership programs with UW Extension, which provides support services to the program and students, while the CON provides administrative leadership and the required regular and substantive engagement with students.

The UW extension has already offered diverse support for the creation of the Flex Option BSN, such as providing the template for the online learning platform and instructional design services; coordinating admission and collection of fees; designing the financial aid administrative system, and hiring an ASC dedicated to nursing. The UW Extension created a pre-enrollment assessment for students to "self-assess" their ability to be successful in this type of self-directed, learning platform. There were expenses associated with the development and launch of the Flex Option BSN including faculty time for creating the courses, assessments, and modules, as well as instructional design work done by CON staff. UW Extension provided the start-up funds to the CON, to cover development, and continues to cover ongoing expenses to run the program. As enrollment grows, the revenue exceeding expenses will be shared between the CON and UW Extension. A special assistant to the provost was assigned to act as the conduit between UWM and UW Extension.

In addition to the CON launching the flexible BSN, two other programs on campus committed to flexible options: the bachelor of science in diagnostic imaging within the College of Health Sciences and the bachelor of science in information science and technology within the School of Information Studies. The coordination of these three launches required the program leads in each of these schools to work very closely together to address start-up issues, to problem solve, to support each other in pre-launch activities, and to share solutions. In addition to the support received among Flex program leaders, students are encouraged to take supplemental competency sets (courses) through other programs, as appropriate. For example, UW offers freshman- and sophomore-level classes in the flexible format that Flex BSN students can take to complete general education requirements.[15]

Perhaps some of the most important strategies for student success were offering an ASC and the use of proactive, intrusive advising. Students begin the process with a learning assessment, predictive of their likelihood of success with a self-directed, competency-based program. Once this assessment has been successfully completed and the student has been admitted, the student then has immediate access to the ASC. The ASC connects with each student to review transcripts, to set a plan of study, to facilitate enrollment, and to answer questions. The student very quickly learns the role of the coach, including how to contact both the ASC and faculty when needed. The ASC, although currently hired and trained through UW Extension, spends time on the UWM campus, getting to know all of the faculty involved in the nursing competency sets, understanding the curriculum, and keeping communication lines open. Open communication was particularly important at the launch of the Flex Option, as the ASC was hired in Madison, 100 miles away from campus. Initially, we at the CON had to insist that the ASC spend time on OUR campus in Milwaukee, two to three days/week. Now that the program has been accepting students for two years, less time on campus is required for the ASC, as many of the initial issues have been worked out. There still is regular communication between the ASC and the program director and course faculty. All new ASC hires spend time on our campus working with our advisors and the program director.

The success of the Flex Option relies on regular and substantive interaction between the student, the faculty, and the ASC. *Regular* means that the interaction is frequent, consistent, and not initiated solely by the student. *Substantive* means that there is an opportunity for relevant and significant discussion of the academic subject matter content with which the student is engaged in completing. The ASC initiates contact with the student. The student then initiates communication with faculty by submitting a goal-setting assignment (GSA) within the first 10 days of the competency set. The faculty must then reply to the GSA within three to five days to provide feedback. The student will update their GSA within the first 10 days of the second and third month of their three-month enrollment, again with a faculty response. The faculty member then provides regular and substantive feedback on assessments, usually within 72 hours but always within our three to five working day time frame.

The GSA is not optional as it is a requirement of the UW Flexible Option program to satisfy Title IV financial aid regulations of the US Department of Education.[16] Agencies that award financial aid as well as accreditors want to ensure that competency-based education programs, like the Flex Option, provide "regular and substantive student-faculty interaction."[16] If a student fails to complete the GSA, the registrar will drop the student from the set on day 11.

Although the first contact the student makes is with the ASC, students can reach out to faculty members by email for academic issues. Faculty members are encouraged to reply to students' email concerns within 24-48 hours. Students who seem to not be progressing, or who are not submitting learning assessments, are contacted, initially by the ASC with follow-up by the faculty member as needed. Often it is a personal issue affecting the student, and not one that a faculty member can or should manage. The ASC can work with the student to refer to appropriate resources.

This attention to detail at every level contributed to a successful visit from the Higher Learning Commission (HLC) in June 2015, which recommended approval of the Flex Option, specifically citing the regular and substantive engagement between faculty and students in the program (personal communication between the Higher Learning Commission and UWM Chancellor Mark Mone, June 24, 2015).

OBSTACLES AND RESOLUTIONS

The launch of the Flex Option hit many bumps, some anticipated and others encountered along the way. A number of those obstacles are presented here, in no particular order, as all were substantial "bumps"—in data management systems, financial aid, remote proctoring, use of textbooks and graders, online learning platforms, and personnel.

- We quickly discovered the electronic system used by the registrar to enroll, register, and enter grades for students was based on a traditional semester system. The registrar, working with UW Extension, resolved these issues, but none were simple fixes.

- Financial aid became, and continues to be, a concern, as competency-based education clears federal hurdles. While we have been able to access federal financial aid for our UW Flex Option students since November 2016, we had to work with our hospital system partners to help them understand the Flex Option so that their nurses would be eligible for employer-offered financial aid for credits earned in a non-traditional format and schedule.

- Consistency among sets was found to be an issue that was readily resolved by implementing a standard template and common ground rules. Individual assessments that were based on quizzes and exams required proctoring to ensure test security. Finding a proctor service that would be available 24 hours/day, on essentially one-day notice, proved to be an insurmountable obstacle. After many failures, we eliminated all quizzes and exam assessments that required proctoring. This actually proved to be an opportunity for our faculty to create better, more meaningful assessments than multiple choice quizzes and exams.

- There was much discussion about required textbooks. Students were expected to determine their own needs for resources and we were sensitive to the cost of the sets. To advertise a set as being $900, and then to add on required textbook costs, seemed counter-intuitive. After considerable thought about this issue, faculty made the decision to require one nursing textbook per competency set and provide additional open resources for each set. Many true CBE programs do not have textbooks and encourage use of open educational resources, but our faculty curriculum developers felt that they needed a nursing text to guide student learning and focus the assessments. This approach may change in the future, but for now, we have a required text for each set. We also have many additional resources for each competency set—and the student can choose to buy the textbook (or not).

- We initially thought that faculty could develop competency sets and that we could then hire "graders" to follow rubrics for each assessment. We determined that we did not want to pursue this, as graders could not provide the level of substantive interaction as a faculty member with that subject area of expertise.

- We launched the Flex Option within the state, as there were no issues with the state Board of Nursing for post-licensure programs. We did have to notify the board of our decision to launch, and we did notify our accrediting body, CCNE, of the substantive change in a delivery option, which was accepted.

- As the initial launch started slowly, enrollment and set coverage were done through overload payments to faculty, who accepted competency set assignments on top of their current workload. While this provided a source of additional income, as enrollment increased, the faculty moved Flex sets into workload, which eliminated overload payments and acknowledged the time faculty were putting into their sets and students.

- The online learning platform, D2L (Desire to Learn), was one with which faculty were very familiar since it had been used throughout the UW System for residential courses, yet its use for CBE stretched the platform beyond its limit. Both UWM and UW Extension quickly decided to dedicate one instructional designer/media support person from within UWM to this learning platform, and to work with UW Extension on ways to program D2L so that it worked better with Flex programs. That reprogramming was critical to the mission.

- Finding the right ASCs and model for advising was an initial hurdle that we quickly resolved. The original ASC model envisioned coaches working remotely. At UWM, we have a strong student affairs department and know with certainty that the role of the advisor is critical to student success. For the advisor to be successful, he or she must be embedded within the team. CON and UW Extension modified the ASC model so the ASC could work on campus with us two to three days/week. While this was another mission critical step at the beginning, now that the program is running smoothly, it is less of a need. That said, it is still vitally important that the ASCs are well-known to program faculty, and work well with our student affairs advising team and the program director.

CONTINUED CHALLENGES

Although we are now entering our third year with the Flex Option, there continue to be challenges that have yet to be resolved, such as barriers related to federal financial aid regulations. We hope to allow students to be registered for Flex competency sets while being enrolled simultaneously in traditional learning modes, both on campus or online, but dual enrollment is expressly forbidden in current federal Title IV regulations. In a modern form of education, we should be making it easy for students to move seamlessly between educational modalities (online, face-to-face, flexible options) as long as the students make progress toward their learning goals. UW Extension leaders are actively working to get these regulations changed.

FUTURE

The goal is to scale up the Flex Option to nurses who are licensed in states outside of Wisconsin borders. As of January 24, 2017, we made the decision to admit nurses licensed in the contiguous state of Illinois to the UW Flexible Option BSN completion program. Some states require Board of Nursing approval for all nursing programs, while others do not require approval for post-licensure programs. This means for every state into which we consider expansion, we must remain cognizant of state requirements, which seem to change without notice. Scaling is also unpredictable, and we must consider the implications of such expansion on faculty workloads and resources. There are costs associated with advertising and expansion. Wisconsin's funding for higher education has provided challenges to our ability to hire additional faculty as needed. We will scale slowly, on a state by state, basis.

We have also begun assessments of student learning, most recently completing an evaluation of critical thinking in competency-based and traditional online learning environments. Assessments of both the program and student metrics will be ongoing.

Lastly, the CON is facing a scheduled accreditation visit this coming fall 2017. The Flex Option will be part of this visit, as the accreditors look at all our academic programs. We are confident in our program, our ability to explain the Flex Option, and the status of the UW Flexible Option as a national leader in this area. While we expect scrutiny, we also expect successful accreditation.

SUMMARY

CBE has been successfully developed and implemented for many different educational programs. The Flex Option at the University of Wisconsin-Milwaukee is the first of its kind in a public institution for post-licensure BSN completion.

ACKNOWLEDGEMENTS

The authors thank Dr. Julie Sebastian (University of Nebraska Medical Center) for her thoughtful review of earlier versions of this paper.

REFERENCES

1. http://www.brighthorizons.com/~/media/83038b9625e2438cad336879c35c fd14)

2. Institute of Medicine. The Future of Nursing: Leading Change, Advancing Health. (2010). Retrieved January 23, 2017 from www.iom.edu/Reports/2010/ The-Future-of- Nursing-Leading-Change-Advancing-Health.aspx.

3. Aiken LH, Clarke SP, Sloane DM, Lake ET, Cheney T. Effects of hospital care environment on patient mortality and nurse outcomes. *J Nurs Admin.* 2009;39(7-8 Suppl);S45-51.

4. https://www.hrsa.gov/advisorycommittees/bhpradvisory/nacnep/Reports/ sixthreport.pdf

5. http://nursecredentialing.org/Documents/Magnet/MagOverview-92011.pdf

6. Sussman A. Job-seeking nurses face higher hurdles as hospitals require more advanced degrees. *The Wall Street Journal*, October 14, 2015.

7. Duffy M, Friesen M, Speroni K, et al. BSN completion barriers, challenges, incentives, and strategies. *J Nurs Admin.* 2014;44(4):232–236.

8. Sarver W, Cichra N, Kline M. Perceived benefits, motivators and barriers to advancing nurse education: Removing barriers to improve success. *Nursing Education Perspectives.* 2015;36(3):153–156. doi:10.5480/14-1407.

9. http://bsnathome.com

10. http://wcwpds.wisc.edu/related-training/mandated-reporter/resources/adult_ learning.pdf

11. Knowles MS. *The Adult Learner: A Neglected Species.* Houston: Gulf Publishing Co. 1973 (Revised edition 1990).

12. http://www.aacn.nche.edu/education-resources/BaccEssentials08.pdf

13. http://www.aacn.nche.edu/news/articles/2011/11enrolldata

14. http://www.uwex.edu/about/

15. https://flex.wisconsin.edu/degrees-programs

16. https://ifap.ed.gov/dpcletters/GEN1423.html

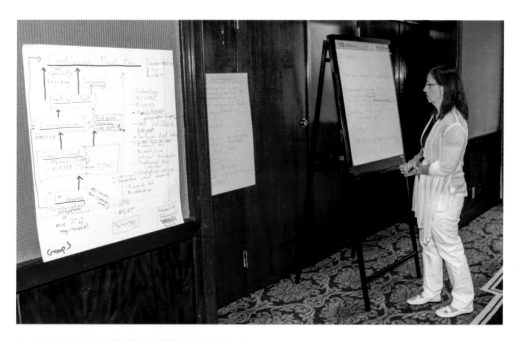

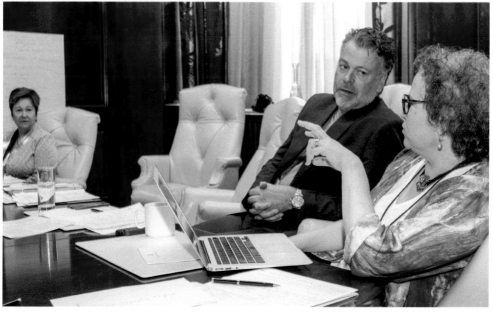

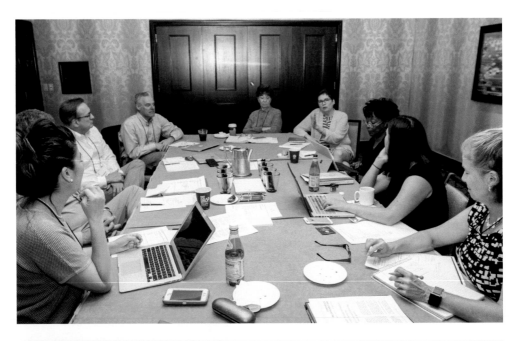

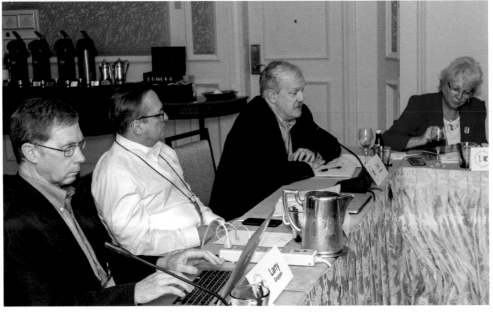

DESCRIBING THE JOURNEY AND LESSONS LEARNED:

IMPLEMENTING A COMPETENCY-BASED AND TIME-INDEPENDENT UNDERGRADUATE MEDICAL EDUCATION CURRICULUM

Case Study

George C. Mejicano, MD, MS, FACP
Professor of Medicine and Senior Associate Dean for Education
Oregon Health & Science University School of Medicine

Tracy N. Bumsted, MD, MPH, FAAP
Associate Professor of Pediatrics and Associate Dean for Undergraduate Medical Education
Oregon Health & Science University School of Medicine

INTRODUCTION

This paper describes a journey that is taking place in Portland, Oregon. The School of Medicine at Oregon Health & Science University (OHSU) has deliberately embarked on a transformation of its undergraduate medical education (UME) program from a classic curriculum to a novel one that is both competency-based and time-independent. For decades, OHSU's curriculum included two years of study focused on basic and behavioral sciences, followed by two years of experiential learning focused on the clinical sciences. In 2012, the medical school began its journey to completely change the UME curriculum to better prepare physicians of the future and to do so in a manner that would embrace a competency-based, time-independent framework.

OHSU did not start this journey in a vacuum. Indeed, most American medical schools had considered, begun, or completed significant curricular changes. The reasons for this were myriad: the limitless explosion in medical knowledge; the emergence of new disciplines such as informatics and genomics; the focus on patient safety and quality improvement; the adoption of new pedagogical formats such as flipped classrooms; decreased public funding for institutions of higher education; the entry of digital natives into the health professions; and the profound impact of legal and economic pressure borne by health care delivery systems and payors.

In response, thought leaders across the country called for fundamental changes in medical education in order to meet the evolving needs of society.[1-3] The literature increasingly championed efforts to incorporate health systems science, teamwork, and interprofessional collaborative practice; to better incorporate technology and high-fidelity simulation into the educational arena; to harness the promise of big data; and to implement curricula and assessment systems that would be based upon learner achievement as opposed to simply time spent engaged in learning.

CONTEXT AND LOCAL ENVIRONMENT

OHSU is the only academic health center in Oregon and is home to numerous research centers and institutes; five health sciences schools and colleges; and a health system comprised of two teaching hospitals, numerous ambulatory facilities, and an integrated faculty practice plan that delivers both primary and tertiary/quaternary care. The university has over 16,000 employees and is considered a public corporation that functions like a private institution even though it receives a small amount of state funding each year, i.e., 1% of a $2.8 billion total budget. The academic centerpiece of the university is the School of Medicine, which is home to 2,032 full-time faculty members, 842 house officers, 570 medical students, and 819 graduate students. In 2016, OHSU was ranked 32nd out of 139 medical schools in the Blue Ridge Institute for Medical Research academic rankings.[4]

In 1995, the medical education program changed its curriculum so that preclinical students would interact with patients in primary care settings. Despite this advancement, the curriculum still consisted of a traditional "2 plus 2" model. The first two years housed nine discipline-based, basic science courses in addition to a "doctoring" course that included a longitudinal preceptorship. The last two years were divided into a traditional third year (i.e., rotations through seven core clerkships that predominantly involved inpatient experiences) and a fourth year that required a sub-internship; a critical care rotation; clerkships in neurology, a surgical subspecialty and ambulatory pediatrics; and 18 weeks of electives.

Two months after a 2012 site visit by the Liaison Committee on Medical Education (LCME) the school's dean charged a team of administrators, faculty, and staff members to transform the UME program. Shortly thereafter, the School of Medicine recruited one of the authors of this paper (GCM) into a new position as the senior associate dean for education. Both authors of this paper served on the team that would eventually be known as the school's curriculum transformation steering committee (CTSC).

The CTSC spent six months exploring different models of medical education before coalescing on a set of guiding principles that would guide the development of a transformed curriculum. The guiding principles incorporated ideas such as the importance of being learner-centered; the need to foster critical thinking, inquiry and lifelong learning; the provision of opportunities to individualize learning; the integration of basic, clinical, and health system sciences; the promotion of active learning; and a commitment to competency-based education. Importantly, the CTSC articulated that the new curriculum's goal was to effectively prepare graduates for residency training and professional practice to best serve and meet the needs of society in the 21st century.

Just as the guiding principles were being socialized to a wide array of stakeholders, members of the CTSC became aware of a grant opportunity that would serve to jumpstart the efforts being envisioned. Namely, the American Medical Association (AMA) released a request for proposals as part of the landmark *Accelerating Change in Medical Education* initiative: 10 schools would each receive awards of $1 million to help bring their ideas to fruition. The authors and a small writing team began to explore nascent ideas that promised to extend the curricular changes already being planned into a full-fledged competency-based, time-independent model. A proposal was submitted in the spring of 2013 and OHSU was awarded the grant a few months later.

The impact and importance of this award cannot be overstated: it brought in external resources and convened a cadre of like-minded colleagues across the country who formed a consortium of thought leaders in medical education. Most importantly, it validated the ideas and concepts being considered by the CTSC. One year later, further momentum was achieved when OHSU was selected by the Association of American Medical Colleges (AAMC) to be one of 10 schools to participate in the *Core Entrustable Professional Activities for Entering Residency* pilot.

 Although the CTSC would continue to meet for another year, Dr. Bumsted—who had been recently appointed as the new associate dean for undergraduate medical education—turned her attention to implementation of the ideas that had been articulated and approved. She convened a development team—consisting of scientists, clinicians, educators and staff—who focused on further developing the new foundational phase of the curriculum. This team determined course goals and objectives and mapped them to the six domains of competency championed by the Accreditation Council for Graduate Medical Education (ACGME). Meeting weekly, the team also worked on organizing content into a series of seven integrated courses (blocks) connected by longitudinal threads, created objectives at the level of individual sessions, mapped the curricular content and articulated the general framework of the foundational phase of the curriculum.

As the development team was finishing its work and prior to launch, an operations team was selected. This operations team comprised approximately 50% development team members and 50% new members, and had responsibility for leading the new blocks and threads, delivering content, and creating assessment instruments aligned with the framework set forth by the development team. A similar process was used for creating the new clinical experience phase of the curriculum (i.e., a development team focused on concepts was followed by a different group that was responsible for implementation).

The new curriculum, called *YourMD*, was successfully launched in August 2014. It consists of two phases. The first focuses on foundational basic, clinical, and health system sciences and typically lasts 18 months. The clinical experience phase consists of clinical rotations interspersed with intersessions (i.e., new, two-week courses that integrate basic, clinical, and health system science content related to four important topics facing society), as well as dedicated time for completion of a scholarly project. Students can explore electives at any time during the clinical phase of the curriculum, e.g., they can rotate in a dermatology service without first having to rotate in traditional experiences such as internal medicine or surgery.

In addition, all medical students are assigned a coach who guides the creation of individualized learning plans that effectively customize students' curricula to meet their interests, who prepares them for their chosen specialty, and who helps improve their academic performance. The coaches have access to a home-grown electronic portfolio called the OHSU Research in Evaluation Data for Educational Improvement (REDEI) platform, which allows tracking of each student's academic progress, including all the data associated with assessment.

Graduation requirements include passing three US medical licensing examinations (USMLE); completion of a scholarly project; passing an interprofessional course focused on patient safety and collaborative practice; successful completion of transition courses; a summative clinical performance examination; and participation in required and elective clinical rotations, including rural and clinical continuity experiences. Clinical experiences in seven core disciplines are required, unless (a) the student obtains a waiver signed by a clerkship director, their coach, and the Associate Dean for UME or (b) the clerkship offers a pathway to bypass the requirement through direct assessment.

To obtain a medical degree from OHSU, students must demonstrate that they have achieved a documented level of competence, (i.e., a specified milestone) across 43 distinct competencies. This is analogous to demonstrating their ability to perform at level 1 milestones described by the ACGME.[5] Students must earn digital badges that signify that the school has made a summative determination of entrustment for all 13 core entrustable professional activities (EPAs) for entering residency described by Englander and colleagues.[6]

WHAT HELPED?

National Events and Issues

First, OHSU performed an institutional self-study in the fall of 2011 as part of the re-accreditation process. The LCME shared its findings with the school in 2012 and this helped create a sense of urgency because the medical education program was found to have numerous elements that were non-compliant or that needed monitoring. The fact that an accreditation agency had uncovered problems "softened the ground" and sent a very strong message that there was much room for improvement.

Second, the successful grant proposal to the AMA led to validation of ideas, granted permission to innovate, secured external resources, and provided an opportunity to network with innovators at the national level. Similarly, the selection of the program to participate in the *Core EPAs for Entering Residency* pilot program sponsored by the AAMC led to further validation of ideas, even more permission to innovate, and a broader network of innovation colleagues.

The final force that helped was the roll out of the ACGME's Next Accreditation System in 2014. This national system embraced the concept of milestones and competencies as cornerstones of how post-graduate trainees must be assessed and tracked over time, and it supported the role of using a competency-based framework in UME. Since competency-based systems rely on workplace-based assessment, the ACGME's emphasis on the clinical learning environment highlighted for us the importance of aligning our efforts with the needs of OHSU's health care delivery system.

Supportive Stakeholders

Change could not have occurred without the support and buy-in from institutional leaders, e.g., the university president, the university provost, and the medical school dean. Indeed, the dean had directly fostered the curriculum change process by charging the CTSC, pushing for rapid deployment of the changes envisioned, recruiting change agents, securing internal resources, and fostering a culture that embraced the principle that the school existed to serve society.

Another set of key stakeholders was a group of junior faculty who were "waiting in the wings," eager for opportunities to participate in the curricular transformation. Whereas faculty who had held leadership roles or had great influence in the old curriculum were sometimes hostile to the ideas being brought forth, dozens of junior faculty members supported the changes being considered. Indeed, senior faculty were surprised that so many people were willing to help the transformation. A final group of stakeholders were prospective students who were eager to join in on something new. These trailblazers were attracted to an innovative curriculum. This also surprised some skeptical senior faculty members who erroneously had predicted a drop in applicants to the UME program because of the curriculum transformation.

Available Resources

We were fortunate to have both internal and external sources of funding. The internal funds were secured by positioning the curriculum transformation as a capital project. Similar to a building project, the new curriculum was framed as a strategic investment that required funding separate from the operational budget needed to run the previous curriculum.

Other resources included individuals at OHSU with specific skill sets in education such as curricular mapping and faculty development. The luxury of having well-respected educators with credibility and national reach proved highly valuable. A related resource included faculty champions who spoke out in support of the changes. The influence of these individuals was far reaching. Finally, OHSU was fortunate to have new and improved learning spaces that opened just as the curriculum launched. These included a new collaborative life science education building with flexible learning spaces, state-of-the-art technology, and brand new simulation suites ideal for interprofessional learning.

Local Circumstances

The development team met weekly and had room to brainstorm ideas before implementation began. Expansion of the class from 132 to 153 students per year helped provide funds because of increased revenue from tuition. It also forced growth of new clinical training sites that proved invaluable in overcoming political opposition at some of the traditional training sites. Another important local factor was the governance by which the school operates. Specifically, both the curriculum committee and faculty council allowed approval of the guiding principles, curricular concepts, competencies, and grading policies in small packets. Relatively low-stakes voting allowed progress to occur without having to burn valuable political capital.

Finally, a major campus-wide initiative that helped people think outside the box was the OHSU Interprofessional Initiative. This initiative required a change in the academic calendar so that the medical students could learn about, from, and with students in the dentistry, nursing, pharmacy, nutritional science, and physician assistant programs. Further, the Interprofessional Initiative required faculty development related to new and more effective instructional methods. Most importantly, this initiative forged communication and collaboration amongst the faculty that eventually helped create consensus on nine interprofessional competencies that all academic programs at OHSU embraced. Traditional barriers such as dissimilar academic calendars, disparate learning goals, and false assumptions about other professions were overcome. Full implementation of the vision of interprofessional education and collaborative practice remains a work in progress, but faculty have enjoyed the opportunity of working and teaching together in an interprofessional manner.

Effective Change Management

The Kotter model was deliberately chosen and selectively utilized to help drive change.[7] For example, the dean as well as the school's communications team used the technique of creating a "burning platform" for change on a regular basis. Similarly, small victories were celebrated so that momentum could be maintained.

Throughout the journey, stakeholder engagement was used to socialize ideas and obtain buy-in to concepts and ideas. One example of engagement involved faculty and student teams that worked together on specific issues, e.g., technology in the classroom, integration of the sciences, program evaluation, student assessment, faculty development, and teaching methodology. Other examples included a school-wide kickoff retreat, surveys to elicit broad input into planning, communication with alumni, road trips to communities across the state, and town halls and small group discussions with faculty and health system leaders. An ongoing and deliberate campaign was utilized to reinforce important messages and garner support. Numerous communication modalities were used to generate enthusiasm including podcasts, videos, print materials, web pages, and social media.

Another change management strategy was the deliberate utilization of key opinion leaders external to OHSU. These included prominent medical educators invited to the campus to discuss changes occurring across the country. Similarly, hosting a national meeting of the *Accelerating Change in Medical Education* consortium provided ample opportunity for internal stakeholders to hear and see what other innovations were being implemented by other schools. This exchange of ideas continues to this day because a steady stream of visitors want to see first-hand what we have done. Similarly, OHSU teams have visited five other medical schools and several faculty members have participated in Harvard-Macy program courses.

In contrast to the safer methods described above, two other change management strategies that were used carried some risk. One of these involved deliberately embracing the uncertainty associated with launching the curricular changes without having all the details of the full transformation finalized. A second one involved the rapid speed of change because the dean had set an ambitious implementation timeline. Some faculty members thought changes were taking place without much forethought despite the rationale that had been communicated by curriculum leaders. The combination of an unwavering commitment to change and the speed of deployment made effective resistance difficult to muster.

WHAT HINDERED?

Regulatory Issues

In contrast to the forces that helped foster change, there also were formidable factors and issues that hindered our progress. These included regulatory issues, reluctance and resistance, and local circumstances. The first occurred in the summer of 2012 when the LCME issued a warning to the school about the medical education program. Although the findings helped create a sense of urgency, they came with a price, because time and energy had to be spent addressing several long-standing problems. In addition, LCME's Element 6.8 states that "a medical education program includes at least 130 weeks of instruction,"[8] setting a minimum standard that constrains any accredited medical school interested in instituting time-independent curricula. Similarly, time-independent medical education programs that would allow graduation to occur throughout the year may find a challenge with the National Residency Match Program's (NRMP) "all-in" policy that requires registered residency programs to attempt to fill all positions through the match only once a year.

Another important factor that hindered progress in implementation was a series of "Dear Colleague" letters from the United States Department of Education. These documents provided guidance to institutions of higher education interested in creating competency-based academic programs. The content of those letters included, but was not limited to, the following:

- The distinction between credit hour competency-based education and direct assessment;

- Requirements for establishing credit hour equivalencies in direct assessment programs;

- Requirements for regular and substantive interaction between students and faculty;

- Prohibition on paying Title IV aid for credit earned through prior learning assessments;

- Satisfactory academic progress;

- Return of Title IV funding provisions; and

- Accrediting agencies' roles in reviewing competency-based education programs.

Because aid eligibility is linked with university accreditation, some campus officials at OHSU have had concerns that implementing a competency-based system might lead to the university losing its ability to provide federal financial aid to enrolled students.

Reluctance and Resistance

The faculty and students had other issues and concerns. First, a cadre of well-respected, senior faculty members opposed the proposed changes. Some concerns raised by these individuals were deeply felt and were brought forth with good intentions. Other concerns were frankly based upon fear of losing power, control, and resources at both the individual and departmental levels.

Particularly troublesome were the chairs, vice-chairs, and other key opinion leaders of entrenched departments. Some of these powerful individuals fought tooth and nail to preserve the status quo. This has been aptly described in at least one peer-reviewed article as the challenge of "curricular ossification."[9] Faculty members who assumed that their personal curricular influence would be preserved were shocked by the loss of "time on stage;" the perception that their subject matter may have lost some of its luster; a perceived loss of reverence for their expertise; and the requirement to attend faculty development sessions designed to incorporate active learning methods. A few of these individuals openly critiqued the changes by stating that OHSU was bound to produce subpar physicians because the new curriculum was "MD light." Certain faculty members experienced professional loss and seemed to go through a grieving process akin to the five stages described by Kubler-Ross.[10]

Another group involved staff in the registrar's office, as well as staff in the financial aid office. These individuals feared that implementing a competency-based, time-independent curriculum would lead to an increase in workload because of the increased complexity associated with tracking students' progress toward graduation, difficulty in changing the transcript, and the cost of re-programming the software used to monitor enrollment and updating financial aid models.

Individuals associated with graduate medical education (GME) programs also raised concerns. Residency program directors did not want OHSU to switch to a "pass/no pass" grading system for clerkships. Skeptical about the use of untested competency-based assessments, they voiced concerns that they would have to increasingly rely on students' USMLE scores to determine the annual NRMP rank lists.

In contrast, student resistance was sporadic and was verbalized most keenly by the last cohort to experience the prior curriculum. By and large, students supported the changes envisioned. However, members of the Class of 2017 occasionally expressed a sense of being neglected because so much attention was focused on the changes taking place. Interestingly, students who have experienced the new curriculum have a different concern: they want to be heard and have their feedback taken seriously to affect change and make further improvements. Thus, a number of feedback systems have been put into place to accommodate this need, including monthly town halls, frequent meetings with administrators, and posting what the UME program has done as a result of the feedback, i.e., "You said; We did." In addition, two new student affairs deans have been hired to improve support for our students and proactively address their questions and concerns, as well as help manage the uncertainty that is inherent with any change of this magnitude.

Finance officers in the school also raised some objections because of the costs associated with implementation and operating a competency-based system. Faculty development, computer systems, new facilities, and "buying protected time" for coaches and course directors require significant and sustained use of resources that would otherwise be spent on other initiatives. Lastly, nearly everyone was concerned about change fatigue and how much faculty time and effort were needed to implement the new curriculum in a successful manner.

Local Circumstances

With regards to the local environment, numerous other challenges surfaced. For example, the departmental compensation model for educational effort was historically linked to "faculty time on task" as well as the number of credit hours associated with each course and clerkship. It was no surprise to hear that a new curriculum that re-organized content, emphasized new concepts such as health system science, and allowed acceleration would result in angst, fear, and uncertainty. In contrast, the authors were caught off guard by the fiery response that occurred when a rumor spread that falsely suggested that the school would no longer require its medical students to participate in a rural clerkship. This was triggered when powerful stakeholders in the Oregon legislature were immediately notified that changes to the rural clerkship were being considered following an internal meeting with clerkship directors.

In fact, the school and its educational leaders never wavered from this commitment. Rotating in a rural setting remains an important graduation requirement. In contrast, what did change was a decision that allowed the rural requirement to be fulfilled by participating in an expanded array of specialties and rural experiences, e.g., rural surgery or working on a community project in a small town could both take the place of a traditional rural rotation involving primary care. The furor that was unleashed by the rumor included student protests, online petitions, calls into talk radio shows, faculty meetings, two state-wide listening trips, the creation of a rural medicine advisory board, and discussion about the UME curriculum in the Oregon legislature. In retrospect, we could have—and should have—anticipated this type of resistance and mitigated its effect given the longstanding importance of rural medicine to the state.

Progress to Date

All in all, the factors supporting change outweighed the factors favoring the status quo. A decrease in resistance has continued since the curriculum transformation was launched in 2012, and there has been much progress in implementing a competency-based, time-independent framework.

First, the faculty and administration conceptualized, and articulated, an end product for the UME curriculum: residency-ready learners that will better serve society. Second, the guiding principles—including the commitment to have a curriculum that is competency-based—were approved without controversy. Forty-three new competencies organized into six domains were approved. Behavioral descriptors (i.e., milestones) are being used to help determine whether a student has performed at a level commensurate with what is expected on their first day of residency. The school has also adopted the 13 core entrustable professional activities (EPAs) for entering residency as a graduation requirement.[6]

The assessment process has been centralized within the dean's office and grading in all phases of the curriculum has been standardized. Grades given to students in the foundational phase of the curriculum are pass, but not yet pass/fail. Toward this end, we have built in real-time remediation options for students who initially do not meet the passing threshold for any foundational block. If they pass their remediation assessment, which covers only their areas of deficiencies, they pass and progress so they can continue with their cohort. This is possible because we have structured a one-week period known as "enrichment week" that occurs at the end of each foundational course, where students needing to remediate can consolidate their learning and attempt to pass a remediation examination one week later. In this example, the student is considered to "not yet have initially passed" the course but can still achieve a passing grade if they subsequently pass the remediation assessment(s). Students that do not need to remediate use this time to explore areas of interest and attend scheduled activities that enrich their learning.

We are still working to solidify our approach to competency assessment in the clinical clerkships. As such, students currently are simultaneously graded along two parallel tracks: a traditional method with tiered grades (i.e., A-B-C-D-F) based upon their clerkship performance through the lens of a specific discipline, in addition to a pass/not yet passed, competency-based assessment that relies upon observation of behaviors associated with one of three levels: pre-entrustment, approaching entrustment and entrustment for a given competency. Each clerkship has a minimum of four competencies linked with it, and these are selected by the clerkship director as those that can be taught and assessed during that rotation. Of note, this means that there is no restriction to a student taking a clerkship multiple times to achieve entrustment for a given competency. The program has also designated a required number of entrustment judgments needed for each competency, e.g., six qualified assessors must attest that a student has achieved entrustment to be judged as passing a specific competency at the programmatic level.

Thus, students graduating in 2018 and beyond not only must pass their required clerkships, but also must accumulate a specified number of judgments that document that they have been deemed to have achieved a pre-determined level of behavior ("entrustment milestone") across each of the 43 required competencies. Starting in summer 2017, summative decisions will be made by a UME entrustment group using a model that is comparable to the clinical competency committees in GME.

Another success has been the creation of the REDEI electronic portfolio that houses assessment data for each student. Trained academic coaches have protected time to meet with students and help them develop individualized learning plans that incorporate student interest as well as track progress in meeting graduation requirements.

Health system science has been integrated into the curriculum. In the foundational phase of the curriculum, a clinical case of the week helps frame the content being taught and the students must access a learning "sandbox" using the health care system's electronic health record. In other words, students begin to learn how to use a key component of the modern health care system—an electronic health record—as they are learning the foundational basic and clinical sciences, beginning in the first week of medical school.

In addition, digital badges have been designed and will be used to display in the REDEI portfolio whether and when a summative decision about entrustment has occurred for each of the 13 core EPAs for entering residency. These digital badges will have a two-year lifespan because the faculty have determined that summative entrustment decisions should be time-limited and specific to each EPA. Lastly, to optimize learning in GME, information about (a) competency level achieved and (b) entrustment decisions made will be forwarded to residency program directors before post-graduate training begins.

Standardization of the clinical experiences has also provided students with the flexibility to explore their interests very early in their career. This is possible because the required core clerkships are all four weeks long and they do not have to be taken in sequence. Thus, a student interested in urology could schedule an elective rotation in April of their second year of medical school, after they have completed the four-week core surgery clerkship, but before they have taken any of their other required core clerkships. One hallmark of a true competency-based system is that students are assessed relative to a standard and not relative to their peers or a given cohort. We have worked to help educate faculty regarding this concept, since previously they would only have had fourth-year students in their electives.

We have created a new course entitled "Transition to Clinical Experiences" and have modified significantly an existing course entitled "Transition to Residency." These courses incorporate many hands-on activities, instruction, and simulation-based assessments. They are also both considered to be "gateway" courses that help determine whether students are ready to enter their next phase of training.

Time-Independence

OHSU, to date, has had less success in incorporating processes that will make the curriculum time-independent. Some of this lack of progress is a result of curricular design. For example, an organ-system focus in the foundational phase of the curriculum integrated content from many disparate fields. An unforeseen complication of that design is that medical knowledge is a domain of competency that is difficult to unpack into discreet components. For example, a student with expertise in physiology cannot easily test out of a foundational course because the content also includes anatomy, public health, microbiology, professionalism, etc.

Thus, the decision to integrate many disciplines has made acceleration through the foundational phase difficult unless one can bypass the *entire* 18-month foundational phase of the curriculum. Nevertheless, there is evidence that acceleration is possible because OHSU admits two dentists in each medical school class as part of the university's oral and maxillofacial surgery program (OMFS). Before starting medical school, these individuals have obtained their dental degree and have also taken the comprehensive basic science exam ("mock USMLE Step 1 exam").

The UME program provides these OMFS students a ticket for the Step 1 examination. In turn, they immediately schedule the exam and receive the results approximately three to six weeks after starting medical school. If a passing score is achieved, a high-stakes clinical skills examination is scheduled to ensure that these students can safely enter the clinical experience phase of the curriculum. If this clinical skills examination is passed, the students take the Transition to Clinical Experience course and then accelerate directly to their clerkships in October of their first year of medical school (i.e., they have accelerated through 18 months of the curriculum in approximately 8 weeks). To date, all six OMFS students who have attempted this pathway have passed both the USMLE Step 1 examination and the school's high-stakes clinical skills examination, demonstrating that acceleration is possible for a select group of students.

Another step toward time-independence is that OHSU has a process that allows students to skip certain required clerkships. To date, 78 students have accomplished this by passing a National Board of Medical Examiners shelf exam and demonstrating competency in performing a history and physical examination for the neurology clerkship. However, thus far, no students have obtained a complete waiver of a clerkship through the process of obtaining the required three signatures described earlier.

We also have developed a pilot program entitled Oregon Family Medicine Integrated Rural Student Training (Oregon FIRST): students interested in specializing in family medicine and practicing in a rural environment may spend nearly their entire fourth year of medical school in Klamath Falls, Oregon, a rural community that is home to an OHSU family medicine residency program. One to two students per year are selected for this program. The purpose of Oregon FIRST is to create a pathway for select students to seamlessly transition into their residencies. In addition to completing required clerkships and electives in this system, they have a longitudinal clinical experience where they develop their own patient panel. Assuming the students match into the Klamath Falls Family Medicine GME program, they will take care of the same cohort of patients in their continuity clinic during residency. Once the assessment system is fully implemented, it is anticipated that Oregon FIRST students will graduate from medical school and begin their family medicine GME program whenever they are deemed "residency-ready" during that year.

Finally, we have engaged over 60 faculty, staff, and learners in the design of a new OHSU Program to Accelerate Competency-based Education (PACE). Students selected into this pilot program will be able to enter an OHSU residency program in a wide variety of disciplines outside of the match. Because OHSU's academic calendar is based on quarters, students can earn their MD degree four times a year. Therefore, we envision that PACE will allow entry into OHSU residency programs approximately 4 weeks after the end of each academic quarter. The group working through the legal, logistical, conceptual, and political issues involved with PACE are in the process of addressing approximately 80 questions that have been identified about implementing such a program.

OHSU Healthcare supports nearly 270 GME slots because the hospital is well over the federal cap set by the US Centers for Medicare and Medicaid Services. Since the university directly supports these residency positions using clinical revenue, we have the luxury of being able to reserve GME slots for students in the PACE program. In this manner, OHSU Healthcare will be able to support students who start their residencies off-cycle. However, this program will likely require an exemption from the NRMP to comply with the "all-in" policy. We anticipate that PACE will be implemented with the medical school class that enters in 2018, and that approximately 16 students will become residents well before the rest of their classmates.

We acknowledge the financial issues associated with a time-independent program. However, we consider this issue to be an opportunity and not an insurmountable challenge. For instance, an important decision we made is a commitment to reduce the cost of the MD degree. Thus, if students graduate early, they will owe less tuition compared with their peers who take the standard four years to obtain their degrees. Indeed, one outcome we are tracking is the overall level of student indebtedness because debt will decrease when students graduate early. However, this will be offset to some extent by tuition revenue from a proportion of the class that graduates later than expected because they have not met their competencies or EPAs to be entrusted as "residency ready."

Although the overall vision to fully implement a competency-based, time-independent curriculum has not yet been realized, steady progress has occurred and the ultimate goal is to have a program that has the following additional characteristics:

- Rolling admissions and matriculation to the medical education program;

- Ability to customize each student's curriculum in a manner that (a) considers past experience, demonstration of knowledge and skills, and each student's interests; and (b) is based not on time spent learning, but rather only upon the results of rigorous assessment and fixed degree requirements; and

- Graduation when the student has demonstrated the requisite skills and that they can be entrusted by the program to safely enter their next phase of training.

LESSONS LEARNED

The OHSU School of Medicine did not start this journey with the goal of implementing a competency-based, time-independent UME program. Rather, the school's educational leaders believed and continue to believe that such a framework strongly supports the goal of creating better prepared residents. Along the way, we have learned several lessons that may be helpful to others considering a similar journey of implementing a competency-based, time-independent curriculum. These are summarized below.

- Start with the end in mind. This fostered a sense of pragmatism and allowed the school to take an innovation approach.

- In the words of Voltaire, "do not let the perfect be the enemy of the good." Implementing components and phases as soon as they were developed helped overcome resistance and sustain forward momentum.

- Maintain an unwavering commitment to stated principles. This served as a constant reminder of why we had embarked upon the journey.

- Know when to compromise. We recognized the value of receiving input from interested stakeholders, encouraged continued engagement, and demonstrated our receptivity to a wide range of ideas.

- Perseverance and grit are essential. Anyone embarking on such a journey should expect ups and downs, good days and bad days, wins and losses, etc. because changes of this magnitude do not come easily.

- Tolerate risk. This allowed implementation to occur rapidly and diminished the likelihood of getting bogged down in details that would stymie progress.

- Expect resistance. This helped us keep focus and minimize distractions; understanding Rogers' diffusion of innovation[11] helped administrators and faculty leaders weather many storms that arose during implementation.

- Choose leaders wisely. The importance of identifying and selecting people who will transform the vision into reality cannot be overstated; similarly, persistently negative personalities should be politically sidelined as early as possible.

- <u>Effective communication through a variety of channels is critical to success.</u> Meeting frequently with the school's communication staff allowed sharing of ideas, explaining of decisions, and obtaining of feedback to generate enthusiasm and garner widespread support.

- <u>Encourage innovation in a protected and unfettered environment.</u> Many corporations have "skunk works" teams separated from operational duties and production lines precisely because day-to-day issues overwhelm creative problem solving.

- <u>Know how things get done at your institution.</u> In-depth knowledge of governance structures, policies, and procedures was critical to success; careful attention to <u>how</u> change occurs within the institution is just as important as focusing on <u>what</u> needs to change, if not more so.

Finally, our greatest learning is that despite the efforts involved in change management, it is possible to achieve major curricular transformation in a school with an existing faculty and student body. Thus far, every indication is that we can achieve not only a competency-based curriculum that will produce better physicians, but also a time-independent one that will result in a better experience for students and facilitate their progression through the continuum of medical education.

ACKNOWLEDGEMENTS

The authors thank Dr. Stephen Schoenbaum (Josiah Macy Jr. Foundation) for his thoughtful review of earlier versions of this paper.

REFERENCES

1. Irby DM, Cooke M, O'Brien BC. Calls for Reform of Medical Education by the Carnegie Foundation for the Advancement of Teaching: 1910 and 2010. *Acad Med*. 2010;85(2):220–227.

2. Skochelak SE. A Decade of Reports Calling for Change in Medical Education: What Do They Say? *Acad Med*. 2010;85(9):S26–S33.

3. Albanese M, Mejicano G, Gruppen L. Perspective: Competency-based medical education: a defense against the four horsemen of the medical education apocalypse. *Acad Med*. 2008;83(12):1132-1139.

4. Blue Ridge Institute for Medical Research. Total NIH Awards to each Medical School in 2016 including Percentage of Direct and Indirect Costs. Accessed online on March 5, 2017: http://www.brimr.org/NIH_Awards/2016/NIH_Awards_2016.htm

5. Holmboe ES, Edgar L, Hamstra S. The Milestones Guidebook Version 2016. Accessed online on March 5, 2017: http://www.acgme.org/Portals/0/MilestonesGuidebook.pdf

6. Englander R, Flynn T, Call S, et al. Toward Defining the Foundation of the MD Degree: Core Entrustable Professional Activities for Entering Residency. *Acad Med*. 2016;91(1):1352–1358.

7. Kotter JP. *Leading Change*. Boston: Harvard Business Review Press; 1996.

8. Liaison Committee on Medical Education. *Functions and Structure of a Medical School*. 2016. Accessed online on March 5, 2017: http://lcme.org/publications/

9. Abrahamson S. Diseases of the Curriculum. *J Med Educ*. 1978;53:951–957.

10. Kübler-Ross E. *On Grief and Grieving: Finding the Meaning of Grief through the Five Stages of Loss*. Simon & Schuster Ltd; 2005.

11. Rogers EM. *Diffusion of Innovations* (3rd ed.). New York: Free Press of Glencoe; 1983.

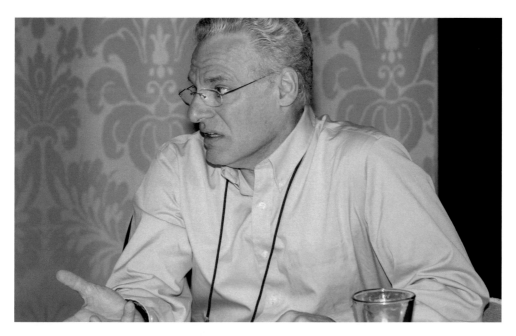

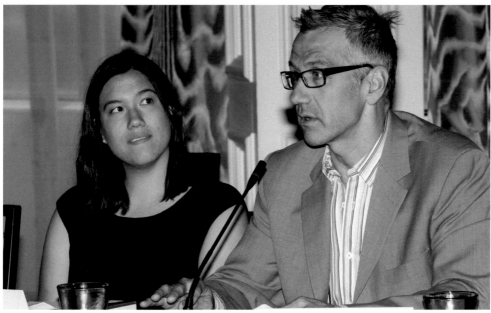

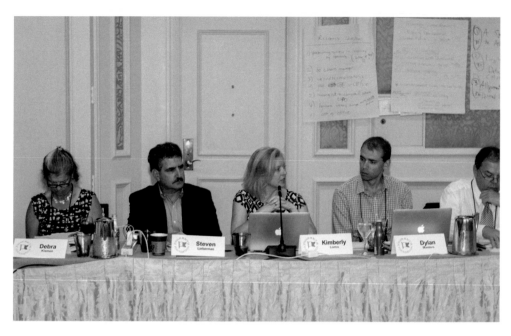

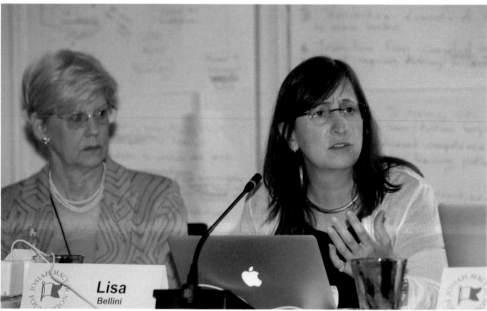

EDUCATION IN PEDIATRICS ACROSS THE CONTINUUM (EPAC):

REALIZING THE DREAM OF TIME-VARIABLE, COMPETENCY-BASED ADVANCEMENT IN MEDICAL EDUCATION

Case Study

Robert Englander, MD, MPH
Associate Dean for Undergraduate Medical Education
University of Minnesota Medical School

Spoiler alert: just as competency-based education is about beginning with the end in mind, we begin with the dramatic ending to this story. *For the first time in North American history, over the 2016–2017 academic year, six students have transitioned from undergraduate medical education (UME) to graduate medical education (GME) based on the demonstration of competence in a time-variable fashion.* These students are part of a remarkable demonstration pilot entitled "Education in Pediatrics Across the Continuum" (EPAC), and we hope the reader will find the telling of the journey to this remarkable conclusion informative and compelling.

THE PROJECT IN A NUTSHELL

EPAC is a national project sponsored by the Association of American Medical Colleges (AAMC), supported from 2013–2016 by a major grant from the Josiah Macy Jr. Foundation, and designed to test the feasibility of advancement from UME to GME, and from GME to practice or fellowship, based on the demonstration of competence rather than time spent learning. Each year for the past three, four pilot sites have chosen two to four students sometime between the end of their first year and the beginning of their third year of medical school who are interested in a career in pediatrics and willing to stay in their home site for residency to experience a continuum of education and training. Each site agreed to recruit at least four cohorts of students and follow them through to graduation from residency.

The core idea of the project is that these students will then advance from UME to GME based on being entrusted to perform the 13 core entrustable professional activities for entering residency (CEPAER)[1] without direct supervision and completing other school-related graduation requirements. Likewise, they will move from GME to practice or fellowship after being entrusted to perform the 17 general pediatric entrustable professional activities (EPAs) without supervision.[2] One important note: this is not a project designed to curtail the length of education and training. While one outcome in moving to a competency-based system may well be a decrease in the *average time* to complete education and training, invariably some learners will take longer than the currently prescribed time to reach the desired outcomes. The focus is on time variability, not shortened duration.

As noted above, six students have already made the first transition in a time-variable fashion, so we are well on our way. The journey to get to this point, however, in a time- and tradition-based world of medical education and training, was not without trials and tribulations. The lessons learned along the way, we hope, will serve the education community as we all try to move to a paradigm in which the outcomes are guaranteed, which by definition means the time to outcomes is variable.

BACKGROUND

Toward the turn of the 21st century, medical education began to take a distinctly new path away from the structure/process model outlined by Flexner in 1910,[3] and toward an outcomes or competency-based paradigm,[4] driven primarily by the Accreditation Council for Graduate Medical Education's (ACGME) outcomes project.[5-6] Around 2008, Deborah Powell, then dean of the University of Minnesota Medical School and upcoming chair of the board for the AAMC, began to have crucial conversations, including a critical one with Carol Aschenbrener, then executive vice president of the AAMC, about developing a model in which the outcomes of education and training were fixed but the time to those outcomes was variable and dependent on a learner's demonstration of competence.[7]

Dr. Powell envisioned a pilot in which students would decide early in their medical school career which specialty they desired, and then advance through medical school to residency in that specialty and, ultimately, through residency to practice or fellowship based on the demonstration of competence in a time-variable fashion. Dr. Aschenbrener agreed to partner with Dr. Powell and the journey toward realizing true competency-based medical education began.

GETTING TO A GO-NO GO DECISION (2010)

Engaging a Specialty Partner

With the AAMC on board, Dr. Powell sought a specialty partner that would satisfy two criteria: a specialty and its leadership poised for educational innovation and medical students whose initial desire to enter the field tended to be static over time. The American Board of Pediatrics (ABP) had just completed a four-year self-study project entitled "Residency Review and Redesign in Pediatrics (R^3P)." The major lesson from this project was that "ongoing changes in pediatric health care require a flexible concept of residency education that can adapt to whatever the future holds, which means that both learning and learning about learning must never stop."[8] The sequel to this project was to design and support the Initiative for Innovation in Pediatric Education (IIPE) program.[9] Dr. Carol Carraccio, the director of this initiative, became a natural partner in exploring the possibility of testing the model through pediatrics.

Buy-in from Regulators

The next step required identification of the key regulatory stakeholders whose buy-in to testing the model would be requisite to its ultimate success. Dr. Powell therefore convened a meeting at the AAMC with the chairs of the boards and chief executive officers (CEOs) of the key stakeholder organizations: the ACGME, ABP, and Federation of State Medical Boards (FSMB). The initial meeting generated both excitement and potential challenges, and prompted a second meeting that included the author of this paper and the AAMC's chief health care affairs officer to identify potential concerns at the hospital or system level for time-variable advancement of residents. The outline of a vision for competency-based advancement was enough to convince the respective organizations of the utility of proceeding to recruit pilot schools and beginning to design the program. The FSMB agreed to advocate with the specific state boards once the pilot schools were determined. Finally, the Liaison Committee for Medical Education (LCME), the accrediting body for medical schools in the US and Canada, was notified of the intended project, ultimately approving track status for all sites that went on to recruit students.

ENGAGING PILOT SCHOOLS (2010-2011)

Choosing the first three pilot schools was an easy task, as participants from the initial meetings volunteered their universities. Thus, the first pilot schools were the University of Minnesota Medical School; the University of Colorado, Denver School of Medicine; and one other school, which ultimately withdrew. In all three cases, they began by enlisting the medical student clerkship director and the residency program director at each school to form the core of the site-specific EPAC team. Dr. Powell also met with the program director for pediatrics from the University of Utah who was enthusiastic about the pilot. He pitched the idea to his dean and the University of Utah became the fourth site. These four sites, along with Drs. Powell, Carraccio, Aschenbrener, and two assessment experts from the University of Minnesota, made up the core of the original group that met in the winter of 2011 in Minneapolis.

Following the first meeting, and after agreement to proceed with a planning phase, Dr. Powell spoke to each of the school's deans to ensure buy-in and commitment as this would likely be a long project given the desire to see it through the UME and the GME phases of the formation of a pediatrician. Several months later, Dr. Powell had an exchange with pediatric education leaders from the University of California, San Francisco (UCSF). They were also enthused about the project and joined as the fifth site.

With the five sites in place and on board to begin, Carol Aschenbrener decided that the AAMC would benefit from someone to lead this and other competency-based education projects for the organization, and thus created the position of senior director of competency-based learning and assessment. This paper's author was lucky enough to be offered the role and joined the AAMC in June 2011. Thus, the infrastructure was in place to begin the planning phase of the project.

EPAC DESIGN AND PLANNING PHASES (2011-2013)

Defining Teams, Engaging Consultants

The national cohort of the five site teams, the AAMC leadership, Dr. Powell, Dr. Carraccio, and the consultants quickly established a pattern of twice-annual meetings, fall and spring, with local work accomplished between meetings. The cohort decided that each team would include up to four individuals, at least two of whom had to be the UME and GME leaders in pediatrics (clerkship and residency program directors, respectively). It also identified other valuable consultants, resulting in an ongoing presence from the ACGME, a member of the National Board of Medical Examiners (NBME) for assessment expertise, and Dr. Gail McGinnis and Dr. Jones who had co-led the R^{3}P project, all of whom stayed engaged directly through the planning and early design phase.

Establishing Guiding Principles, Primary and Secondary Goals

One of the first tasks of the cohort was to establish a set of guiding principles that would lead us through this work and serve as a foundation for the many times we knew we would hit barriers over the ensuing years (see List 1). The guiding principles covered the project at large and then aspects of the project related specifically to assessment and faculty development. Once we had established the guiding principles, we turned to the development of primary and secondary goals. After much debate, we decided that we were first and foremost a feasibility study for competency-based, rather than time-based, advancement across the continuum of education and training. We also realized that we would need to demonstrate no harm as a result of this pathway, and that the pathway might have the opportunity to mitigate some of the harm created by the traditional fragmented rotation-based (rather than relationship-based) education and training. We arrived, therefore, at the following primary goal:

> The primary goal of the Education in Pediatrics Across the Continuum
> (EPAC) project is to establish a model for true competency-based
> medical education through variable-time, meaningfully assessed

demonstration of competence across the continuum of undergraduate medical education, graduate medical education, and independent practice.

We then established the following secondary goals:

1. Do no harm (each student would be in good academic standing, meet all graduation requirements, and have board scores and competency performance comparable to or better than students in the traditional pathway);

2. Improve empathy compared with students in the traditional pathway; and

3. Decrease burnout compared with students in the traditional pathway.

Agreeing on Competency and Assessment Frameworks

To achieve our primary goal meant coming to agreement on the competency and assessment frameworks that would establish readiness to transition from UME to GME and from GME to practice. *This is a crucial point and worth a pause to re-emphasize: If you are going to undertake a competency-, rather than time-based advancement program, then by definition you have to start from a common mental model of the desired outcomes and alignment on how you will assess them!* For the competency framework, we began with a discussion of the ACGME framework, as all accredited GME programs were already using the ACGME competencies and milestones as the basis of their assessment. The difficulty in this case was the wide variation across sites at the UME level regarding institutional expected outcomes or competencies. The AAMC's publication of the "Physician Competency Reference Set" (PCRS) made the standardization easier by aligning directly with the ACGME competencies and providing a single framework for use across the continuum from entry to medical school to exit from practice.[10] While not all schools in the pilot had adopted this framework, we thought we could obtain buy-in, at least for the pilot's purposes, as this framework would provide a continuum that links UME competencies with GME competencies. Thus, all schools would need familiarity with the PCRS as a part of ongoing business with the AAMC. Additionally, most of the competencies from the PCRS aligned with the pediatric competencies and their milestones,[11] allowing further linkage from UME to GME.

Agreeing on the competency framework was only half the battle. Competency-based advancement would require an overarching framework, standard performance criteria for transitions across the continuum, as well as a core set of assessment tools within a program of assessment adopted across sites. Carol Carraccio introduced us to the concept of EPAs and the group was excited at the prospect.[12-13] For our second meeting in 2012, therefore, we invited Olle ten Cate, who became an ongoing consultant for the project. In retrospect, the decision to go with EPAs as the organizing assessment framework for EPAC was a high-risk endeavor, as there were no UME EPAs at the time and the pediatric EPAs were very much in development. However, knowing that the design phase would require innovation at every turn, the team felt that the EPA concept probably was the most apt to succeed. Thus, as we transitioned into 2013, armed with our guiding principles, our competencies and milestones, and the promise of UME and pediatric EPAs, we were ready to tackle the design phase of the project.

Attaining Alignment within Sites

One of the most important early steps was to make sure that the structures to support the pilot at each site were engaged and aligned. This work included Dr. Powell's reaching out to the deans at each site, and the site teams meeting with their educational leaders and curriculum committees. In one case, the unintended error of omission of the curriculum committee engagement resulted in about a six-month backtracking before the team could proceed. The onboarding of a new vice dean for education who needed to be convinced that the project aligned with her strategic priorities compounded the problem.

The First Major Failure

No pilot project can claim to be successful without failures. Our first major failure came before we even enrolled the first student. In the winter of 2012-2013, one of our pilot sites had to drop out. The root cause was a change in leadership that unearthed an alignment gap. The vice dean for education, who had been the main administrative champion for the project, left the school. The dean, briefly with direct oversight of the project, decided that it was not a priority and withdrew support from his team. Absent support for their time and effort, and given that we had not yet committed to any students, the site team opted to withdraw from the program.

...But Challenges Bring Opportunities

The loss of one of our five pilot sites underscored our notion that we needed to find additional funding or risk losing more sites. We had sought outside funding to supplement the investment of the AAMC from a couple of sources, but redoubled our efforts after the departure of our colleagues. Thankfully, after presenting the idea to the Macy Foundation, we were invited to submit a proposal. Even then, the Macy Foundation saw the potential of a time-variable, competency-based advancement model! The Macy Foundation was also interested in breaking down the UME/GME barriers to create a true continuum as well as the concept of earlier differentiation of learners. The resulting grant of $900,000 over three years ($300,000/year) was a major factor in our ability to move into the design and implementation phases. Of note, every penny of that grant went to support faculty at the sites and protect their time to do the work of design and implementation. Progress on these fronts was made possible only by the continued support of the AAMC for the two meetings per year, the time of Drs. Aschenbrener and Englander, and the consultants required to fill our gaps and complement our skill sets as well as the in-kind support of Drs. Powell (from the University of Minnesota) and Carraccio (from The ABP Foundation).

Overcoming Additional Hurdles

In addition to needing financial support for our sites, the group also struggled with two major aspects of the project: assessment and program evaluation. Despite the best efforts of our core teams and those who were consulting on the project, the "add-on" nature of this work to everyone's busy jobs made progress on assessment and program evaluation difficult. Toward the end of 2012, therefore, the AAMC agreed to support two consultants, one for each of the areas requiring assistance. We were lucky enough to enlist the help of Alan Schwartz, PhD, Michael Reese Endowed Professor of Medical Education at the University of Illinois College of Medicine at Chicago, for our assessment efforts and Doreen Balmer, PhD, then from Columbia University and currently Director of Research on Pediatric Education at Children's Hospital of Philadelphia, to lead our program evaluation efforts. Supporting the time of these highly skilled consultants stimulated rapid advance of the project design.

Getting to Alignment on Assessment

Led by Dr. Schwartz, one person from each site, along with those consultants with expertise in assessment, formed the Assessment Working Group. This group set out to determine how to come to a common mental model of competence and criteria for transitioning from UME to GME and GME to fellowship or practice through an assessment program. We established that entrustment to perform the CEPAER[1] without direct supervision would serve as the foundation for the decision regarding advancement from UME to GME and that entrustment to perform the pediatric EPAs unsupervised would serve as the foundation for the advancement from residency to fellowship or practice.

The sticky issue, then, was how to get to those entrustment decisions in a way that would be equivalent, though not necessarily equal, across sites. The group agreed to adopt a standard set of assessment tools across sites as well as maintain use of selected local tools. After input from Tara Kennedy, a short-term consultant, who advised us based on her expertise in clinical oversight and supervision,[14] the group also agreed to use a supervision scale adapted from Chen et al. as the primary tool for making entrustment decisions.[15] In addition, they agreed to have those decisions made by clinical competency committees (CCCs) based on aggregate data that informed performance on each EPA. They decided to have all 13 of the UME EPAs assessed using this supervision scale, and to take a "deep dive" into the literature for five of the EPAs to piece together valid, evidence-based assessment tools that address the competencies critical to entrustment for the given EPA. Interestingly, while the resultant assessment "portfolios" were to have a core set of shared tools across sites with additional tools based on local preferences, all teams thought they would have a much better and shared model of competence among them than any of them felt they had in the current time-based model.

As we now enter the GME phase of the project, we are in many ways "starting over." Although the EPA framework is the same, the implementation of pediatric EPAs for trainee assessment, integrated with competencies and milestones, began in 2016 at 22 pilot sites (all the EPAC sites are engaged), and so much of the groundwork is yet to be done. The purpose of this pilot is to explore program directors' *a priori* expectations of the level of supervision required for graduation for each of the 17 pediatric EPAs and compare it with actual performance following a cohort of trainees after their three years of residency. The results of this study will help inform transition points from GME to fellowship or practice for EPAC trainees.

One advantage, however, is that the GME programs have been engaging CCCs for a couple of years, and thus the infrastructure for entrustment decisions is in place, whereas this was a *de novo* requirement in the UME portion of EPAC.

Program Evaluation

Led by Dr. Balmer, and joined by a member from each site and consultants with expertise in program evaluation, the Program Evaluation Working Group formed and has begun to define how we will evaluate our primary and secondary outcomes. Dr. Balmer's framework for program evaluation pursues the primary goal of obtaining actionable information throughout the pilot to allow constant course correction, while at the same time making it possible to assess whether we have been successful in our primary and secondary goals.[16] Our first charge, therefore, is identifying the enabling and disabling factors that affect feasibility. We are accomplishing this through site visits (by Dr. Balmer) and data gathering yearly from each site at large and at each of the twice-annual meetings from the team members (including students). Additionally, to test our secondary hypotheses, we are measuring empathy and burnout in our cohort and controls, matched for an interest in pediatrics (UME), and by residency program (GME) yearly.[17-19]

Readying for Implementation: Recruiting Students

As with other major areas of project development, the national cohort approached the selection of students with the notion that some aspects of the selection process should be consistent across sites and some should be site-specific. For example, early on, the group decided that the entrance timing could be variable. As a result, the sites vary from entry at the end of the first year to entry in the early part of the third year of medical school. This allows us to look at some of the factors affecting feasibility. For example, does earlier entrance to a program that requires career specialty identification and commitment to a specific site for residency result in more dropouts (due to an ultimate decision that pediatrics is not the right fit or a compelling reason to leave the residency catchment area)? Conversely, does late entrance curtail the interested pool of applicants, making recruitment more difficult?

For the common portion of recruitment, the sites agreed on an application process and required that students who are accepted be in good academic standing. As this is first and foremost a feasibility project, our goal has been to recruit students whom we think have the best chance of progressing. Ultimately, the ideal would be a lottery system for all students interested in the EPAC program that would allow generalizability of our findings. However, we decided to "stack the deck" at least in the early years to focus on obtaining proof of concept.

IMPLEMENTATION PHASE (2013-2014)

Operational Support

As with any new educational program, the implementation of EPAC required operational support and coordination. Thanks to the Macy Foundation grant, each school hired administrative/project coordination help to augment the faculty leaders' oversight. These program coordinators have been invaluable and all site leaders are clear that the project would be untenable without them. The difficulty has been moving them from grant support to an operational line in the school's budget as the grant has come to an end. All sites have continued support through this year, with three promising continued support next year. If the fourth site loses its administrative support, the consortium will be tested again to come up with new approaches to make sure we can complete our commitment to the active cohort of students.

Regulatory Hurdles

Despite our best efforts to get our "ducks in a row" with the regulatory agencies, we encountered two hurdles through the UME and transition to GME phases. First, California law had a minimum time requirement for UME to allow eligibility for licensure. Because of pressure from EPAC and from UC Davis, another site working toward implementing time-variable advancement, the California state legislature reversed that law and eliminated the time requirement for licensure. Second, the National Residency Matching Program (NRMP), which we kept informed of the project, developed an "all-in" policy, the consequences of which the consequences of which make it difficult to move a student from UME to GME outside the match between the time the rank lists are required from programs (early February) and the end of the academic year. The remainder of the academic year, however, remains open for time-variable advancement.

Financial Hurdles

One major issue that has arisen is what the financial model should be for students who advance early. At the University of Minnesota, for example, students pay for the degree by agreeing to pay for 11 trimesters at the cost per trimester that they pay on arrival to medical school. This is a wonderful arrangement for any student completing the degree in four or more years, but presents a problem for someone completing the degree in, say, 10 semesters. Financial aid implications become salient for students who are ready for transition to residency, but have remaining tuition for which they receive financial aid. In schools with a semester tuition model, what happens to students who are ready to transition at the beginning of a semester? These issues are still being addressed at each of our sites.

Curricular Issues: EPAC Explore, EPAC Focus, EPAC Cohort

As the group got ready to recruit its first cohort, we began to focus on our need to engage and recruit students from arrival to medical school (or even before, as our sites now note the EPAC program as an example of the school's commitment to educational innovation). One of the schools came up with the concept of a program that could match the potential increasing commitment of a student to EPAC, and the other sites have since adopted this construct. On arrival, each site informs students about the project as early as orientation but invariably during the first semester. The sites invite students to join "EPAC Explore" if they think they have an interest in pediatrics and might be interested in the program. During this phase, students have the opportunity to learn with and from pediatric faculty and at times have placements in pediatric settings for shadowing. They also now can get early exposure to the members of the first two to three cohorts. In the next phase, "EPAC Focus," students identify an increased likelihood of applying and get more intensive exposure to the program. This group ultimately provides the applicant pool. These students continue to have additional opportunities in pediatrics. Finally, there is a call for applications from the EPAC Focus group, and each site chooses up to four applicants.

The Clinical Immersion Experience: To LIC or not to LIC?

Early in the program design phase, the question arose as to whether the clerkship model of the third year of medical school could support a competency-based advancement pilot or whether a longitudinal integrated clerkship (LIC) would be superior.[20-21] We consulted the expertise of David Hirsh from Harvard and Kathy

Brooks from the University of Minnesota to help us think through what a specialty-specific LIC might look like, a potentially new undertaking without precedent worldwide. From a logistics standpoint, not all the sites could commit to a LIC for the project, and the EPAC consortium ultimately decided that this could be a variable portion of the curriculum.

As with any variation, our goal will be to try to understand the resultant associations. Is competency-based advancement easier in a LIC than a traditional clerkship model? Is competency-based advancement even possible in a time-based clerkship model? Is there a difference between progression in an EPAC-specific, pediatric-based LIC (as at the University of Minnesota) versus a general LIC with non-EPAC students (as at UCSF)? Despite the site variation, each site committed to longitudinal relationships with preceptors and clinic patients as continuity is one of our guiding principles. Finally, is an EPA framework, with the embedded notion of entrustment, more easily implemented in a LIC with longitudinal relationships with preceptors? [22] While our small numbers will not allow us to get to correlation, asking the questions and looking at the available qualitative and quantitative data should at least inform future research questions.

Attrition

We have had one student decide that pediatrics was not the right choice so far in the three cohorts (entering the program in the 2014-2015, 2015-2016, and 2016-2017 academic years) that are at least partially through their clinical immersion experience. From the outset, we set a number of "opt-out" opportunities. This withdrawal was a good indication that those checks in the system are working.

The Cultural Evolution or Revolution

A revolutionary outcome that seems to be developing is that students are taking ownership of their education and assessment. The traditional mindset of medical students toward feedback may be summed up as students only wanting to hear positive comments or nothing at all, and often wanting to escape the radar. In contrast, EPAC students are self-assessment seekers.[23-24] They approach preceptors about the EPAs they are working on and request observation and critique of their skills so that they can improve. The EPAC students own their education and assessment. They are also often the experts on the expected behaviors for the core EPAs and thus can serve as a resource to the preceptor.

LESSONS LEARNED

The journey to date, from inception to buy-in to design to planning and, finally, to implementation, has resulted in many lessons learned about implementing a time-variable, competency-based advancement system in a predominantly time- and tradition-based model. Key lessons include the following:

- Obtain stakeholder buy-in, especially of regulatory bodies, early in the process, and keep them informed. Any organization whose rules or regulations are invested in the current time-bound model need to be engaged and provide buy-in in advance of the recruitment of students. In our case, that included the LCME, ACGME, ABP, FSMB and each of the relevant state medical boards.

- Obtain leadership buy-in and then follow-up. Any major educational innovation will require the buy-in of the dean and the governing structures of the medical school or residency program (e.g., curriculum committee).

- Agree up front on what the outcomes are and how they will be assessed. What are the desired outcomes that form the basis for your advancement decision and how do you know when they are achieved?

- Consider alternative education funding strategies. Our current strategies are clearly set up for a time-based model of education and training. How can we allow students who demonstrate competency to transition early without penalizing them financially and, likewise, how can they stay when advancement is slower than expected without additional financial burden?

- Empower students. One of the major lessons from this model has been the transformation of students from a focus on auditioning for residency to a focus on becoming great doctors once the pressure of the match has been removed. Additionally, all students note feeling empowered by the clear delineation of expectations and the path to achieving them.

- Relationships matter. The elements of continuity in patient care and longitudinal relationships with faculty preceptors and mentors instill motivation and responsibility in learners. An example of this has been demonstrated by the feedback-seeking behaviors of the EPAC students.

- <u>Resources are key to educational innovation and transformation</u>. Without the initial and ongoing support of the AAMC and the Macy Foundation grant that saw the project through a critical three years, including implementation, the likelihood of success would have been minimal. Innovation takes people and time. The support of the AAMC and the Josiah Macy Jr. Foundation gave national validation to the importance of this work. We are equally certain that their support will add credibility to the outcomes.

NEXT STEPS

EPAC is in its eighth year since Dr. Powell first approached Carol Aschenbrener at the AAMC with a hope and an idea. Our third cohort either is chosen or is about to be chosen at our four sites and several students have already made the time-variable transition from UME to GME. Despite these successes, there is still so much to do and learn. For the current and future cohorts, can the two schools that have not yet done so advance future cohorts in a time-variable fashion? If not, what are the impediments? What seem to be the critical factors for success?

We are just entering the GME phase, and so will ask and study the question: did time-variable progression work? Do the EPAC residents perform at least as well or better on the pediatric milestones and EPAs as their non-EPAC counterparts? Can we advance learners through residency based on competence rather than time? What does a time-variable transition from GME to practice or fellowship look like? What are the licensing and accrediting implications that we have not yet thought of?

Once the four cohorts have been chosen, what will happen at our sites? Will there be a fifth? Will the programs continue even after the national pilot is complete and the AAMC is no longer acting as the "glue" holding the project together? How will sites convert these programs from innovation to operations? Finally, in addition to continuing to learn and grow within EPAC, if the project continues to have successes, we need to consider scale. What is the next specialty that could/should try the EPAC model? How can the program be expanded to other pediatric sites?

While there are many questions left unanswered, one thing is certain: *For the first time in North American history, over the 2016-2017 academic year, six students have transitioned from undergraduate medical education to graduate medical education based on the demonstration of competence in a time-variable fashion.* And that's a story worth telling!

ACKNOWLEDGEMENTS

The author thanks Dr. Carol Carraccio (The American Board of Pediatrics) for her thoughtful review of earlier versions of this paper.

REFERENCES

1. Englander R, Flynn TC, Call S, et al. Toward defining the foundation of the MD degree: Core entrustable professional activities for entering residency. *Acad Med.* 2016;91:1352–1358.

2. Carraccio C, Englander R, Gilhooly J, et al. Building a framework of entrustable professional activities supported by competencies and milestones to bridge the educational continuum. *Acad Med.* 2017;92:324–330.

3. Flexner A. *Medical Education in the United States and Canada. A Report to the Carnegie Foundation for the Advancement of Teaching.* Boston, MA: Updyke; 1910.

4. Carraccio C, Wolfsthal S, Englander R, et al. Shifting paradigms: From Flexner to competencies. *Acad Med.* 2002;77:361–367.

5. Swing SR. The ACGME outcome project: Retrospective and prospective. *Med Teach.* 2007;29:648–654.

6. Swing SR, Beeson MS, Carraccio CL, et al. Educational milestone development in the first 7 specialties to enter the next accreditation system. *J Grad Med Educ.* 2013:98–106.

7. Cooke M, Irby DM, O'Brien BC. *Educating physicians: A call for reform of medical school and residency.* San Francisco, CA: Jossey-Bass; 2010.

8. Jones MD, McGuinness GA, First LR et al. Linking process to outcome: Are we training pediatricians to meet evolving health care needs? *Pediatrics.* 2009;123(S1):S1–S7.

9. Carraccio C, Englander R. IIPE: The Path Forward to Transforming Pediatric Graduate Medical Education. *Pediatrics* 2010;125:617–618.

10. Englander R, Cameron T, Ballard A, Dodge J, Bull J, Aschenbrener C. Toward a common taxonomy of competency domains for the health professions and competencies for physicians. *Acad Med.* 2013;88:1–7.

11. Carraccio C, Gusic M, Hicks P (editors). The Pediatrics Milestone Project. *Academic Pediatrics.* 2014;14 (2 suppl):S13–S97.

12. ten Cate O. Entrustability of professional activities and competency-based training. *Med Educ.* 2005;39:1176–1177.

13. ten Cate O, Scheele F. Competency-based postgraduate training: Can we bridge the gap between theory and clinical practice? *Acad Med.* 2007;82: 542–547.

14. Kennedy TJT, Lingard L, Baker GR et al. Clinical oversight: Conceptualizing the relationship between supervision and safety. *J Gen Intern Med.* 2007;22:1080–1085.

15. Chen HC, van den Broek WES, ten Cate O. The case for use of entrustable professional activities in undergraduate medical education. *Acad Med.* 2015;90(4):431–436.

16. Bolman L, Deal T. *Reframing organizations: Artistry, choice and leadership* (3rd ed). San Francisco: Jossey- Bass; 2003.

17. Maslach C, Jackson SE. The measurement of burnout. *J Occupational Behavior.* 1981;2:99–113.

18. Hojat M, Gonnella JS, Nasca TJ et al. The Jefferson Scale of Physician Empathy: Further psychometric data and differences by gender and specialty at item level. *Acad Med.* 2002;77:58-60.

19. Hojat M, Mangione S, Kane GC et al. Relationships between scores of the Jefferson Scale of Physician Empathy (JSPE) and the Interpersonal Reactivity Index (IRI). *Med Teach.* 2005;27:625-628.

20. Ogur B, Hirsch D, Krupat E, Bor D. The Harvard Medical School - Cambridge integrated clerkship: An innovative model of clinical education. *Acad Med.* 2007;82:397-404.

21. Gaufberg E, Hirsch D, Krupat E, et al. Into the future: patient-centredness endures in longitudinal integrated clerkship graduates. *Med Educ.* 2014;48(6):572-582.

22. Englander R and ten Cate O. LICs and entrustable professional activities: A perfect match. IN Poncelet A and Hirsh D (eds) *Longitudinal Integrated Clerkships: Principles, Outcomes, Practical Tools and Future Directions*. North Syracuse, NY: Gegensatz Press: 2016.

23. Watling C, Dreissen E, van der Vleuten CPM, et al. Learning culture and feedback: an international study of medical athletes and musicians. *Med Educ.* 2014;48:713-723.

24. Eva KW, Regehr G. "I'll never play professional football" and other fallacies of self-assessment. *J Contin Educ Health Prof.* 2008;28:14-19.

LIST 1. EPAC GUIDING PRINCIPLES

Framework for Curriculum and Assessment/Evaluation

1. EPAs for a general pediatrician are the framework for the program. These EPAs are mapped to the domains of competence and competencies, and their corresponding Pediatric Milestones providing a clear linkage for learners and faculty.

2. In addition to meeting the school and LCME graduation requirements, subsequent transition points (UME to GME and GME to fellowship or practice) will be contingent upon meeting the predetermined thresholds for transitioning within this program as follows:

   - Learners will meet expected levels of performance for milestones and levels of entrustment for designated core EPAs

   - Learners will bring a "portfolio" of individual learning needs at transition points.

3. Learners, teachers, and the learning environment have a shared responsibility in achieving program and individual goals.

4. Advancement according to demonstrated ability that results in entrustment will be the primary criteria. Learner progress in the program must be based on performance against specified outcomes (the competencies as demonstrated through certifiable or entrustable activities), not only on time.

5. Learner assessments will be performed using tools and processes common to all EPAC sites and tied to the Pediatric Milestones supplemented by assessment tools required by individual schools for their curriculum.

6. Learners are both empowered and expected to be key participants in their own assessment.

7. Qualitative and quantitative data about programs and learners will be collected longitudinally and shared with the consortium.

8. Learners will be required to pass all components of USMLE in accordance with USMLE guidelines.

9. The curriculum must cover the breadth and depth required by the LCME.

Continuity of Experience

1. Continuity of relationships will be an organizing principle of this pilot. As such there must be continuity of relationships with faculty, other students in the cohort (locally and nationally), the interprofessional health care team, and patients over the continuum of training to ensure relationship building, role modeling, mentoring, and the degree of direct observation essential for entrustment.

2. Learners must have longitudinal experiences as part of the health care team that allows them to follow patients in a meaningful role over time, with progressive responsibility and entrustment for care.

3. Learners should be able to develop a comprehensive understanding of the development of health and disease throughout the life cycle and through the lens of a future pediatrician, (e.g., through an understanding of the childhood determinants of many adult diseases and the implications for prevention).

Logistical Considerations

1. Each program site must allocate residency positions for learners to enter when they meet the requirements for the UME-GME transition.

2. Each site must allow re-entry to existing traditional MD program for learners who decide to opt-out. This will be done in time to allow completion of other traditional pre-residency requirements. Each site must accommodate voluntary leave of absence during the training period as required by the LCME or ACGME.

3. Learners should be identified and enrolled in the pilot by the mid-point of year 2 but must be enrolled no later than the beginning of the major clinical experiences.

4. The EPAC pilot sites should create a national learning community.

Quality and Safety Considerations

1. Continuity experiences should occur at sites that have demonstrated commitment to continuous improvement of patient outcomes.

2. The program offers a unique opportunity for learners to follow and work on projects to improve the health outcomes for the population of patients that they follow over time. Sites should make this a goal of the program and select health care environments where this can be accomplished.

Faculty Development

1. The program (EPAC) will provide the project team faculty with guidance and support to prepare for the implementation of the project at their sites. The sites will need to provide faculty development in competency-based advancement and assessment, mentoring, etc.

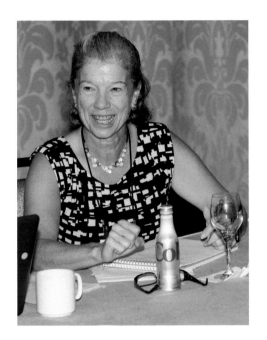

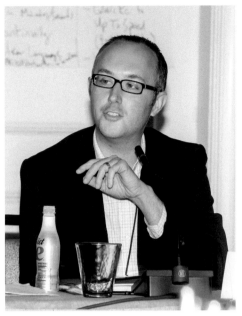

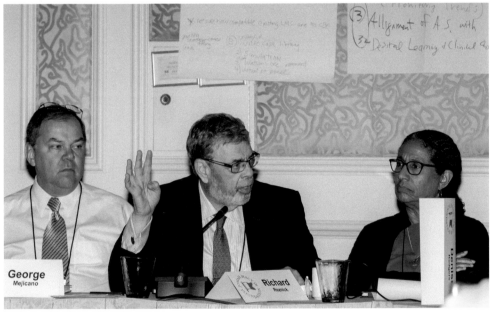

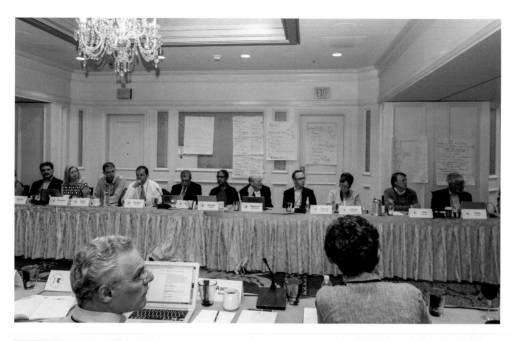

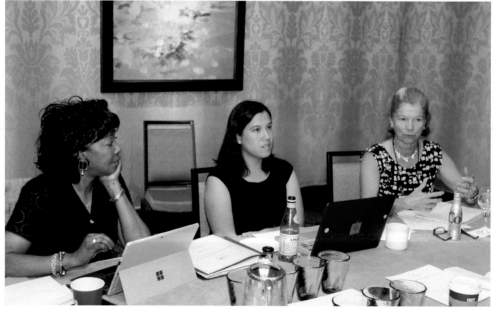

HIGHLIGHTS FROM THE CONFERENCE DISCUSSION

The educators, administrators, researchers, regulators, medical residents, and others who gathered for the Macy conference on "Achieving Competency-Based, Time-Variable Health Professions Education" engaged deeply in thoughtful discussions, which we have done our best to capture here for readers who may be interested in more details. During the conference, the 39 conferees participated in both plenary sessions and smaller breakout conversations that enabled them to jointly draft, consider, refine, and ultimately agree to a set of recommendations intended to help health professions schools make progress toward educational reforms that will better prepare learners for practice in today's health system. The final recommendations are detailed in the "Conference Recommendations" chapter of this monograph, and below is a day-by-day overview of how the recommendations were crafted by the conferees.

During the first full day of the conference, participants discussed two commissioned papers and three case studies—all of which are included in this monograph—and engaged in breakout groups to prepare for thematic discussions the following day. On the second day, conferees participated in breakout groups organized around major themes, challenges, and opportunities on which to base a set of actionable recommendations and they discussed findings from the breakout groups in a plenary session. At the close of day two, the conference planning committee became a writing committee and drafted preliminary recommendations based on the previous two days of discussion. The final half-day was devoted to achieving initial consensus around the draft recommendations, which were then revised, refined, and finalized via conference calls and emails in the weeks following the conference.

DAY 1: THURSDAY, JUNE 15, 2017

Opening Remarks and Introductions

Following a welcome reception, dinner, and introductions the evening before, the conference began at 8:00 a.m. on Thursday, June 15. During his opening remarks, Macy Foundation President George Thibault, MD, introduced the topic of competency-based, time-variable health professions education (CBTVHPE) by positing a "fundamental" question to conferees: "Is there a better way to produce health professionals that are better prepared to meet the needs of the public? That, to me, is the goal of health professions education and it is what we should be asking ourselves as we discuss this topic." He went on to pose follow-up questions, asking, "is there also a more efficient way—not just a better way, but also a more efficient way—to educate our health professionals? And, is competency-based, time-variable education an answer to these questions?"

Thibault asked conferees to also keep in mind the potential impacts of achieving competency-based, time-variable education on other important health system goals, including whether or not it can help 1) improve the racial/ethnic and geographic diversity of the health professions workforce; 2) expand interprofessional education and collaborative teamwork; 3) increase engagement and partnerships with patients, families, and communities; and 4) impact job satisfaction and personal wellness of health professionals. He also asked conferees to think about the topic in the context of the full continuum of health professions education, from undergraduate and graduate education through professional development and continuing education that spans entire careers. Dr. Thibault enjoined the conferees also to think about scale, asking if CBTVHPE is something that should be for all learners or only some? "These are all cross-cutting issues that I'd like us to be thinking about as we engage in this conversation," Thibault said.

Conference Chair, Catherine Lucey, MD, from the University of California, San Francisco School of Medicine, followed Dr. Thibault's comments, stating, "The real challenge for us is to make sure that our educational programs are sound enough to reliably produce a workforce that is going to ensure that every patient gets the type of care that we would want for someone that we care deeply about." She went on to explain that currently, "We are not 100% confident that everyone who moves through our educational programs—whether in medicine, nursing, pharmacy, dentistry, or social work—is equipped to meet the needs of individual patients and improve the health of entire populations." She suggested this reality as the backdrop to the conferees' conversations about competency-based, time-variable education.

Dr. Lucey also provided a caveat: that quality should be at the forefront of any educational reform efforts. "I believe that [health professions] educational quality has to be measured against similar quality measurements as patient care." This means that CBTVHPE must be safe for learners and for patients alike; it must result in high-value, efficient care; it must be educationally sound; it must be equitable and inclusive; and it must be patient-centered. She also mentioned that time variability in education is not about accelerating or slowing down the amount of time that a learner spends learning, but is instead about "optimizing" the amount of time each learner needs to learn.

Following these opening remarks, two commissioned papers and three case studies were summarized and then discussed by the full group of conferees.

Overview and Discussion of Commissioned Paper:

Time-Variable Training in Medicine: Insights Derived from the Literature and from Examples in Practice

The first commissioned paper, *Time-Variable Training in Medicine: Insights Derived from the Literature and from Examples in Practice*, was presented by lead author, Olle ten Cate, PhD, professor of medical education at University Medical Center Utrecht, in the Netherlands. His co-authors were Eugene Custers, PhD, (University Medical Center Utrecht); Larry Gruppen, PhD, (University of Michigan Medical School); Lorelei Lingard, PhD, (Schulich School of Medicine and Dentistry, Western University, Canada); Pim Teunissen, MD, PhD, (Maastricht University, the Netherlands); and Jennifer Kogan, MD, (University of Pennsylvania Perelman School of Medicine). Upon introducing the paper, ten Cate said he would "cherry pick" a few highlights from it, starting with the fact that the length of time learners have traditionally spent in medical education and training is an "historical given" and not something that was deliberately investigated and decided upon, or for which much evidence exists.

Further, if we look around the world, there are many differences in the lengths of time spent in medical school and residency training. In the Netherlands, for example, undergraduate medical school is set up to last six years post high school, on average, but there is no set time period between matriculation and graduation, and graduates may enter residency at various times during the year. Given this variability around time in medical education, said ten Cate, there is no reason why we should not consider time-variable medical education.

He then added that transitioning to a competency-based, time-variable educational model would necessitate a rigorous approach to assessment to ensure that learners achieve standards of competence. Unfortunately, because of the variety of workplace contexts, workplace assessment, he said, "is one of the most difficult elements of medical training" and we must recognize and address this challenge if there is to be a shift toward competency-based education. He also offered a warning regarding assessment and time variability: because we tend to rank students based on performance, we would need to be careful not to turn time variability into a new method for identifying and ranking the "most time-efficient" students.

Aside from standards of competence, ten Cate suggested additional motivations for moving toward time variability in education. One important factor: time variability allows for individualization and flexibility in educational programming, which in turn supports learners who have varying reasons for spending more or less time on a task or series of tasks. Some may want to spend more time acclimating within a particular set of competencies without necessarily advancing—the authors called this "dwell time"—or some may need to take time off for personal or family reasons. Others may have already have been exposed to the topic and are, thus, able to move on to the next topic more quickly. This room for individualization within the educational plan is important to protect so that time variability does not become time compression (i.e., accelerating through the program becomes more valued than making deliberate progress), which we may be tempted to label as "more efficient."

Another point raised during the discussion: the need to strike a balance between defining competencies that all medical students—or all health professions students—must acquire and those that only some must acquire, such as those who go into pediatrics or psychiatry or another specialty area. This "differentiation" must be considered and balanced with the need for "uniformity" in competencies for all health professionals. A related point was also made: that time variability could allow for earlier differentiation among learners who know their career paths earlier than others and who don't require exposure to a variety of specialties—such as the student who goes to medical school with the goal of becoming a surgeon or a pediatrician.

Following this brief overview of highlights from the paper, session moderators Robert Blouin, PharmD, of The University of North Carolina at Chapel Hill, and Conference Chair Catherine Lucey opened the floor to questions. The first conversation raised the concept of spacing—as in, is it better to focus on learning one skill at a time or on multiple skills that are interspersed over time? Findings from educational research and the practice habits of musicians were raised as responses to this query—both point to sequencing or interspersing multiple tasks over time as likely to be more productive. This may be different, though, depending on the level of learner (new, expert, or in-between) and the difficulty and complexity of what is being learned.

This led to a comment about the differences in the health professions' approaches to education; specifically, the intermittent nature of nursing education, in which multiple experiences are interspersed, and the more immersive nature of clerkships and residencies, for example, in medical education. This difference points to the need for context when considering time variability in health professions education.

Also raised was the need to assess faculty based on the standardized competencies they will be teaching students and on which they will be assessing students. This marked the first time that faculty development was raised during the conference, but it would become an important theme that threaded throughout the discussions—the recognition that faculty will require support as they transition from traditional teachers in a time-constrained system to student coaches and assessors in a time-variable system. Another issue for faculty is that competency-based assessment—which implies that student attainment of objective competencies will automatically result in good health professionals—may impact both their own abilities to use judgment in the face of uncertainty and their ability to teach that judgment skill to students.

Following this discussion, a conferee noted the need to rigorously assess the interpersonal skills of students (and faculty) because they are so closely tied to patient outcomes. The conferee mentioned that, currently, medical schools are reluctant to remediate students who demonstrate a high-level of academic prowess but a low-level of interpersonal skill, which needs to change. Another commenter raised remediation as a challenge in the current time-constrained system, and fears it could become more challenging in a time-variable system, in which some students might be motivated, for the wrong reasons, to move more quickly than they should through certain topic areas. The commenter was struck by the concept of dwell time as an area for more research—specifically, the need to better understand the role that dwell time plays in a health professional's development—that could help offset the need for remediation.

Continuing the remediation thread, one of the health professions students at the conference raised the idea of time variability as a welcome change to the culture of health professions schools. "I think an assessment system where students feel comfortable trying and then re-trying if they need to, without repercussion and with someone saying, 'here are some things to work on,' would be exciting," he said. "It would be a system where students aren't so afraid of failing as they are now. It might set people up for more and better success later." The need for this type of culture change—shifting to more meaningful feedback that health professions students view as valuable—became a recurring theme throughout the conference.

In fact, another conferee picked up the thread and explained that medical students today are about "impression management" because they've been reduced to grade point averages and test scores as evidence that they are doing well in school. "They think they are their scores," she said, "so no wonder they don't want to admit to not knowing something. We need to teach them that the best way to learn is through failure."

Other topics raised during the discussion of the first paper included the implications of competency-based, time-variable education for interprofessional education, and concerns that such an educational system is not feasible given the current reimbursement system in health care.

Overview and Discussion of Commissioned Paper:

Great Expectations: Competency-Based Medical Education from Reality to Vision

Authors Damon Dagnone, MD, MMEd, and Richard Reznick, MD, MEd, both from the Faculty of Health Sciences at Queen's University in Canada, presented their paper, *Great Expectations: Competency-Based Medical Education from Reality to Vision*, on behalf of their Queen's University co-authors Denise Stockley, PhD, and Leslie Flynn, MD, MEd. Dr. Reznick, who is dean of the Faculty of Health Sciences, began the conversation by stating, "We've been talking about competency-based for a long time, probably 20 years. We're here to argue the point: enough talk, let's do." He then briefly described a "seven-year experiment" at Queen's University that shifted the curriculum to competency-based medical education. Reznik and his colleagues embarked on the curricular transformation several years ahead of a national plan, currently underway, to shift all Canadian undergraduate and graduate medical education programs to competency-based education.

Dr. Dagnone, who is an associate professor of emergency medicine and the faculty lead on the competency-based medical education effort at Queen's, offered more details, walking conferees through the steps taken by the school to simultaneously transition 29 medical specialty programs to competency-based education—a process that is working "extraordinarily well." Dagnone said that the wheels really went into motion about three years ago, when they shifted from a planning effort within Dean Reznick's office to implementation across the entire medical school—or as Dagnone said, "we moved from less talking to more doing."

Essentially, a central team or "nerve center" of faculty and administrators coordinates the effort, working together with active committees within each of the 29 medical departments. The central and departmental teams are focused on three areas of activity: 1) curricular reform; 2) a new program of assessment; and 3) implementing entrustable professional activities for entering residency, as defined by Canada's Royal College of Physicians and Surgeons. "We are constantly in an iterative process of strategic planning, communication, learning from, hopefully, small failures, and just constantly gathering information and readjusting," Dagnone said.

Following the authors' brief summary of their efforts, session moderators Debra Klamen, MD, MHPE, of Southern Illinois University School of Medicine, and George Mejicano, MD, MS, of Oregon Health & Science University School of Medicine, opened up the conversation to conferees, several of whom were struck by the very high level of faculty engagement and development that has taken place at Queen's. "Clearly, a lot of work went into winning both the hearts and minds of faculty," said one. Another conferee, who noted the level of faculty involvement—"they are serving as co-creators of this change," he said—was equally impressed by the levels of interdisciplinary and interprofessional collaboration that the reform effort required and achieved.

Reznick followed up on the discussion about faculty engagement with some details about how it has been achieved, including the addition of "medical education innovation" as part of the department heads' annual performance evaluations.

"You have to put your money where your mouth is to do this," said Reznick. "We knew it wouldn't be perfect, we knew it would be hard, but we committed to doing it. And, now our residency program directors are leading the conversations across the country about how to do this within their specialties."

Another theme that arose during this part of the discussion was the need for a value proposition in favor of CBTVHPE. Several conferees noted how helpful it would be to develop a winning argument and/or to clearly define the problem whose solution is CBTVHPE—at least in part. A conferee suggested that patients could help articulate the problem because they are on the receiving end of the care being delivered. "I hope we can push ourselves to think how we could precisely, for our community, define the problem we're trying to solve," she said, "and how we can use our patients to, perhaps, put some interesting color into that."

Dagnone responded to some of the comments by summarizing what he found to be essential to successful implementation. He mentioned the need for a strategic vision that everyone buys into and the need for a clearly defined structure in place for carrying out the vision. He also mentioned that, as faculty lead, he found it very important to listen carefully to every stakeholder. "I just kept reminding myself to shut up and listen, to let them talk, to reflect back to them that I was hearing them, and then asking them to hold me accountable for helping to move things forward," he said. "It really was a process of co-production, a bottom-up process."

Overview and Discussion of Case Study:

The University of Wisconsin-Milwaukee Flexible Option for BSN Completion

The third paper was an overview of the *University of Wisconsin-Milwaukee's (UWM's) Flexible Option for BSN Completion.* Written by Kim Litwack, PhD, RN, FAAN, dean of UWM College of Nursing, and presented by Aaron Brower, PhD, provost and vice chancellor of the University of Wisconsin-Extension, the case study describes UWM's decision to launch, in 2013, a self-paced, competency-based, bachelor of science in nursing (BSN) degree completion option for registered nurses (RNs). "I want to be encouraging to those who are doing this. It's really hard to make changes in a regulatory environment that was built around a certain model that is not a competency-based education model," said Brower. "The financial models are different and the way you fund programs like this are different. Career incentives are different for people working in it. It's all different, so it is important to take it on organizationally, with everyone on board, and not to pursue a 'lone-wolf' model."

He went on to explain the wide variety of CBE models that exist—"from credit-based, course-based, time-based programs to non-credit, non-course, and non-time-based options"—and described the UW Flex Option as a "direct assessment" model which was implemented within the existing College of Nursing and with the existing faculty. The goal of the program is to help more RNs in the state and the country obtain BSN degrees, as recommended by the Institute of Medicine's "Future of Nursing" report.

Brower described a program that is project-based, in which learners design community health projects and are assessed on the competencies they are required to master. "It's not pass/fail," he said, "it is mastered or not yet mastered, and you have to master every competency to move on, which learners can do at their own speed." The program also features individualized support for learners, with "a lot of assessment on the front end, starting with admissions advisors triaging students into different kinds of programs because the Flex Option is not right for every student." Brower went on to describe how "academic success coaches"—highly paid, full-time professional advisors—are assigned to work one-on-one with Flex Option students.

Brower also discussed the importance of planning and structuring the "non-academic" side of a program like this. In the case of BSN Flex Option, UWM offers the curriculum while UW Extension handles all other operations, including marketing, enrollment, transcripts, tuition, financial aid, and more. "It was very important for us to sort out all these details ahead of time," said Brower. "It helped to have a solid business plan, to know how much enrollment growth we needed and over what period of time in order to break even, given all of the resources that went into creating the option."

Session moderator Juliann Sebastian, PhD, RN, FAAN, of the University of Nebraska Medical Center, then opened the floor to questions from conferees, most of whom asked about accreditation challenges. Brower acknowledged that accreditation was tricky and time-consuming to manage, but also that they found accreditors to be open-minded and helpful around innovation. He mentioned that they also found financial aid to be a particularly difficult challenge—so much so that it took about 18 months to sort out.

Overview and Discussion of Case Study:

Describing the Journey and Lessons Learned: Implementing a Competency-Based and Time-Independent Undergraduate Medical Education Curriculum

The next case study, *Describing the Journey and Lessons Learned: Implementing a Competency-Based and Time-Independent Undergraduate Medical Education Curriculum*, details Oregon Health & Science University School of Medicine's (OHSUSOM) experience transforming its traditional curriculum to an innovative competency-based, time-independent curriculum. George Mejicano, MD, MS, FACP, professor of medicine and senior associate dean for education at OHSUSOM, presented the case study, which he wrote with colleague Tracy Bumstead, MD, MPH, FAAP, associate professor of pediatrics and associate dean for undergraduate medical education at OHSUSOM.

Mejicano said that he would walk conferees through the "who, when, why, and how" of his school's curriculum transformation. He first explained the "why," stating that the school changed the curriculum in order to build a better product—in this case, a physician—so that patients will receive better care. "I believe that we've been producing a product that does not meet society's needs," Mejicano said. "This is not about students. It's not about faculty. It's about the patients. They are the 'who' in our paper." He went on to say that the "when" is now. "We have an opportunity now, and we must strike while the iron is hot," Mejicano said.

He then tackled the "how" of OHSUSOM's curriculum transformation. "It's a political process," Mejicano said. "You have to understand that the change process is steeped in culture and personalities and agendas." He said it is also an exercise in "principled pragmatism over purity" and that it is important to "know where you're going" and also how the effort will be sustained over the long run.

Following Mejicano's brief overview, session moderator Steve Schoenbaum, MD, MPH, of the Josiah Macy Jr. Foundation, opened the floor to questions and comments from conferees. The first comment echoed the characterization of the change process as a political process and suggested that focusing on the benefits to patients—rather than placing students and/or faculty at the center—might make for a better case argument. "I think that we risk, by making this an educational reform issue, we risk people not in education seeing this as fluff," he said. "But we've all bought into it because we know, behind the scenes, that this matters to patients. So starting there gives a little more teeth to this whole idea."

A second commenter added that educational reform to create better physicians is about more than benefiting the patients that are seen in academic health centers, but also those patients—members of the public—who live elsewhere. "Part of our obligation is to create physicians, nurses, and other health professionals for folks who live in places that don't have access to care," she said.

Mejicano was then asked to talk about the use of coaches at OHSUSOM—which is similar to the use of coaches in the Flex Option BSN program at UWM. Mejicano explained that OHSUSOM currently employs about 45 part-time coaches that work with their assigned students from matriculation until graduation. "Our coaches are there to provide honest feedback," said Mejicano. "We've found that the best ones come from graduate medical education (GME)—where they are receiving the 'product,' if you will, and know what to look for—and not from undergraduate medical education (UME)." He went on to argue that, rather than building a "firewall" between coaches and assessors, as some schools have advocated, that the lines between them should be blurred, because the coaches know the students best—often better than those making entrustment decisions.

Additional commenters asked Mejicano about his school's maintenance of two grading scales—a traditional tiered scoring system as well as pass/not yet passed grading on competencies. He said that the traditional system was maintained as "scaffolding" while faculty and students get used to the new competency-based system. He also mentioned that, as far as tuition, students who progress through the school at a faster pace pay less tuition than those who move through more slowly. "We thought long and hard about that," he said, "and there are pros and cons, but we decided it was important to bake that [approach to tuition] into the equation."

The concept of feeding learners forward also was raised, with Mejicano stating that his school's plan is to deliver information about each learner to the faculty overseeing that learner's next educational experience. "Faculty preceptors ought to know where to focus their teaching to help each student progress to the next level," he said. A commenter followed up on this: "One of the problems we have is that we train in one system but expect performance in a different one. If we're trying, ultimately, to get to a co-production model, where teams of providers partner with patients and populations, then we need to train people in the model that is closest to that, that best prepares them for partnering. I ask myself is competency-based, time-variable education the model that gets the learner closest to being able to partner with patients? I think that it is, but we have to be able to make that argument."

Finally, a commenter asked Mejicano to respond to the argument that competency-based training is about achieving a minimum level of competency and does not necessarily encourage excellence. Mejicano said he disagrees, stating, "It's a minimum to ensure patient safety, but it's, hopefully, also a scaffold to produce excellence."

Overview and Discussion of Case Study:

Education in Pediatrics Across the Continuum (EPAC): Realizing the Dream of Time-Variable, Competency-Based Advancement in Medical Education

Robert Englander, MD, MPH, associate dean for undergraduate medical education at the University of Minnesota Medical School, authored and presented the final case study, *Education in Pediatrics Across the Continuum (EPAC): Realizing the Dream of Time-Variable, Competency-Based Advancement in Medical Education*. The paper began with a spoiler alert: "For the first time in North American history, over the 2016–2017 academic year, six students transitioned from undergraduate medical education to graduate medical education based on the demonstration of competence in a time-variable fashion." He went on to explain that the students are part of a "remarkable demonstration pilot" entitled "Education in Pediatrics Across the Continuum" or EPAC, which is underway at four medical schools and was the focus of the case study and his presentation.

During his presentation of the EPAC case study, Englander said he had two "big take-home messages" for conferees. The first is that time-variable progression from UME to GME is feasible. He explained that there are three requirements for competency-based, time-variable education: 1) alignment of regulatory agencies before beginning the transition; 2) agreed-upon clear outcomes; and 3) an agreed-upon plan for assessing those outcomes. "You have to agree, at the end of the day," he said, "about requirements and about what knowledge is needed to say a learner has met those requirements."

For his second take-home message, Englander posed the question: "Is it [CBTV education] better than what we have now?" And then answered it: "Based on our experiences so far in EPAC, and based on other experiences that have been published, like the Toronto experience, I think the answer is 'it's probably at least as good, and maybe better, but we have a lot of work to do to figure this out for sure.'"

He went on to highlight some positive experiences and some minor challenges encountered during EPAC. One of the positives he mentioned, for example, was that students in EPAC—who have already decided to pursue pediatrics and know they will transition to residency early—seem to focus more on being a good pediatrician rather than a good student. "They are able to focus from day one on what is required to be a good pediatrician," said Englander, "rather than just a good medical student." Related to this positive is one of the challenges he mentioned: EPAC students are not really part of a medical school class because they finish after their third year, and they are not really part of a residency class because their timing is different there as well.

At this point, Englander asked Dorothy Curran, MD, an EPAC pediatrics resident at the University of Minnesota, to say a few words about her experience with the program. "I think EPAC works because it's not only competency-based, but also time-variable," she said. "Those things are intertwined and it's difficult to separate them. If you were to eliminate time variability then you go back to the old framework of students trying to do well and not being completely honest about their feedback." Related to this, she said, is the benefit of residency matching through EPAC, which also removes learners' incentives to keep up appearances.

"Knowing where I was going for residency made me very cognizant of what it would take to get there and I didn't want to progress too fast. Conversely, faculty knew they would be on the receiving end of me as a resident and had a vested interest in being honest about my progress."

Session moderator Carol Carraccio, MD, MA, of The American Board of Pediatrics, then invited the conferees to join the discussion. One commenter, an emergency medicine physician, noted that, as a medical student, he would have liked the opportunity, as in EPAC, to choose his specialty early because once he decided on emergency medicine that was all he wanted to do. He also said that, once the decision was made and he saw the breadth and depth of his responsibilities, he was in no hurry to move through the relevant requirements.

Another conferee inquired about EPAC's secondary goals of improving empathy and decreasing burnout among medical students—"not something we typically think with potentially accelerated programming." Englander responded that, when designing the EPAC program, they hypothesized that creating a longitudinal educational experience focused on the development of relationships and competency-based advancement could help mitigate a decline in empathy, but it's too early in the program to know the results.

Continuing on the topic of the learners' experiences in EPAC, another conferee mentioned that medical students are "sick and tired" of competing with each other. By setting them up to compete instead against a standard of excellence, as in competency-based education, students learn to focus on the competencies and on delivering patient-centered care, rather than on demonstrating that they're better than other students. And another raised the idea that competency-based, time-variable programs may work better for non-traditional health professions students, such as emergency medical technicians who bring some skills to their health professions education.

Dr. Englander then reminded the conferees that, ultimately, the EPAC pilot will graduate and train approximately 60 pediatricians, which is a small number from which to generalize findings. The program designers, cognizant of this fact as well as of the self-selection bias inherent in the program, were very careful in choosing which outcomes to measure and how to measure them, but the program is still a few years away from being able to report outcomes.

Dr. Thibault wrapped up the EPAC discussion by explaining to conferees the features of the program that led the Macy Foundation to fund it. He said that the program is set up to explore three very important concepts, including competency-based education, blurring the lines between UME and GME, and allowing students to differentiate themselves early—in this case, by choosing pediatrics at the start of medical school. He went on to explain a fourth factor that he discovered later, during an EPAC meeting: EPAC students' attitudes toward evaluation appear to be changing; they welcome evaluation as helpful guidance for improving their knowledge and skills.

Plenary Session Overview: Reports from Breakout Groups and General Discussion of Themes of the Day

Following presentation and discussion of the two papers and three case studies, conferees were assigned to small breakout groups to focus on specific topics and explore themes relevant to possible recommendations. After these groups met, the afternoon plenary discussion featured brief reports from each of the five breakout groups and a general conversation about the primary themes of the conference so far.

Group 1

The first breakout group to summarize its discussion had been asked to articulate the educational, economic, and philosophical case for CBTVHPE and to anticipate how naysayers might respond. The group's reporter opened by suggesting an "elevator" speech that stated, "When learners experience effective competency-based education, patients receive better care today and better care tomorrow." The group also suggested that another argument might be that it is the responsibility of the health professions to "give assurance to society that we are preparing learners to meet 21st century health care needs" and that "fostering professionalism is a mechanism to retain the privilege of self-regulation" within the health professions.

The group also talked about time variability and two themes emerged. The first is that we should begin viewing time as a resource rather than as an intervention, which is the way traditional education views time. When it is viewed as a resource, it is easier to consider varying it depending on need. Second, the group discussed the fact that competency-based education may or may not be time variable, but that overall it is a component of success in health care, not a total solution to all the challenges, but an important partial solution.

The group also discussed some benefits of CBTVHPE. They suggested that it is a "developmental model" that meets learners where they are and empowers them to be more active in their own education. It also empowers faculty to acquire new skills that tap into their own autonomy and self-determination as teachers. They also suggested that it creates opportunities to weave in interprofessional competencies and to align educational and clinical care outcomes, which "really should be one and the same." The group then talked about the potential return on investment being quite high and considered, for example, that society might benefit by gaining better physicians who provide more cost-effective care. The group also discussed the importance of keeping the tone positive; not assigning blame for the current challenges to particular stakeholders; and tailoring the arguments to the right audiences, realizing that different stakeholders have different priorities.

Finally, there was some discussion around whether the conferees should recommend competency-based, time-variable education as a package or if some components can be competency-based but not time-variable or vice versa. No resolution was reached. The answer to that and many other questions about CBTVHPE, the reporter suggested, lies in the ability to accurately gather, measure, and assess outcomes data—a science that must continue to advance.

Group 2

The second breakout group discussed educational enablers, including technology, people, and policies. In terms of technology, the group discussed various learning management systems and how they are evolving as well as the development and use of digital portfolios and dashboards and how these can provide educators with aggregate data about the students. The group also talked about learning analytics programs and the potential for predictive modeling using big data methods to look at learners' patterns and needs, and about various possibilities for capturing data for assessment in the workplace. The group discussed adaptive assessments that allow for real-time performance adjustments as well as simulation, which is demonstrating real benefits. Finally, various group members said they also discussed some of the collaborative efforts, such as Team STEPPS, as well as the potential for using electronic health records (EHRs) as assessment tools. And one member, acknowledging the privacy concerns and other challenges, raised the idea of a national database to track learners from UME into GME and beyond.

In terms of people—or human resources and faculty development—the group's reporter said that the idea of coaches resonated strongly with the breakout group as well as with the larger group of conferees. She also said that faculty development should be customized for new roles that faculty are being called upon to play, including that of coach as well as educational designer and assessor. The group also discussed teams and how to better assess their performance.

In terms of policies and institutional structures, the group discussed the fact that educational enablers are closely related to an institution's culture and that the culture must make room for these concepts to flourish. They talked about coaching—or intrusive advising—as part of the educational design to which an institution must commit. They talked about other educational design components, including active learning, longitudinal experiences, and fostering educational handovers or transitions between different learning phases. They also brought up various forms of conflict of interest, particularly related to the use and sharing of data. Finally, the group discussed the need for the clinical learning environment to be structured in a way that allows learners to develop relationships with other learners, faculty, health professionals, and patients.

At this point, Dr. Thibault raised a question about tying the various educational enablers the group discussed to competency-based, time-variable education. "Will competency-based, time-variable education mean that all these things that already are part of the educational process, or should be, will actually get done, that we'll be more committed to doing them?" A group member responded: "When you break away from the assumption that time-in-seat results in an educational outcome that you want, then it demands that we do things differently. Think about the resources invested in the coaching of college athletes. We have trainees who are doing such high-stakes, important work and we would never dream of putting that kind of support structure around their development. But, by asking ourselves, 'are they truly ready?' then we start looking at it differently and can't not do it any longer."

Group 3

The third breakout group discussed ways to challenge the dominant paradigm in health professions education by redesigning educational systems, transitions, and accreditation strategies to facilitate CBTVHPE. The group's reporter said that, at first, they had trouble getting started, so they began by mapping out the educational process from college through medical school to GME and clinical training to lifelong practice and they decided during the process of mapping the various educational pathways and processes that the nomenclature itself is a barrier. The group decided to recommend that the entire enterprise of competency-based, time-variable education—from its beginnings in UME to the end of a practitioner's career—as "competency-paced medical practice."

The group attempted to name many of the major barriers to changing the nomenclature, including the deeply embedded culture of medical education and practice, the regulatory agencies, the traditional academic calendar, the way credit hours are tied to both financial aid and accreditation processes, and more. But they didn't dwell on the barriers as much as they discussed how to address them. One idea: competency-paced medical practice would enable dynamic e-portfolios to follow practitioners across a lifetime of entrustable professional activities (EPAs). The group discussed harnessing graduate medical education as a way for practitioners to sunset some EPAs and retrain in new ones as a way to refocus their careers. They also discussed the need to decentralize the "maintenance of certification" process to the workplace to take advantage of existing data streams.

The group also recommended reducing the number of transitions in medical education. Currently there are at least three, but some learners go through as many as four or five, depending on how far they take their training. The group recommended eliminating the transition between medical school and residency training to consolidate time and use it more as a resource. Another recommendation: incentivize collaboration and teamwork and de-incentivize competition by eliminating traditional grades and introducing criterion-referenced assessment and ranking. They also suggested tying patient outcomes to the EHR vendors and incentivize them to work with the education and training programs to solve the attribution error problem. The group wrapped up by acknowledging that the idea of competency-paced medical practice won't get off the ground without regulators and accreditors committing to the shift.

Dr. Thibault and several other conferees applauded Group 3's "provocative" proposal to change the nomenclature to competency-paced medical practice, but Dr. Thibault warned against dropping the concept of education in favor of practice only. "This is not just about practice," he said. "This is also about education in order to do something. That 'something' is take better care of patients and maintain our professional competence. I think we need something that combines the two without dropping education." Following this warning, one conferee urged the group to keep the "competency-paced" concept, while a few others expressed concerns about any attempt to change the existing nomenclature because it is well-established and target audiences may be confused by new language.

Before moving on to the next report, a discussion broke out around the feasibility of the group's recommendation to reduce the number of learner transitions in medical education, particularly by eliminating the transition between UME and GME. While many conferees were intrigued by the idea and named a variety of potential benefits, Dr. Thibault raised a conspicuous organizational barrier: that there are only 140 or so medical schools, but more than 800 institutions that sponsor GME training programs—and there is little connection or continuity between them. Also important to note about this discussion: while it focused on a particular transition in medical education, the concept of reducing and/or improving educational transitions is applicable to all health professions learners—including those in nursing and pharmacy—as they move from the classroom into clinical practice.

Group 4

The fourth breakout group was charged with "building a bigger tent" by identifying quick wins and incentives that could convert CBTVHPE skeptics into supporters. The group began by listing the types of stakeholders whose support would be needed. They include accreditors, regulators, licensors, employers, state and national government agencies, deans, GME program directors, students in the traditional model who may feel left behind, new applicants, faculty, and patients. In terms of a quick pitch to these stakeholders, the group proposed, "Competency-based, time-variable health professions education leads to transparency and clarity in evaluation, which allows students and faculty to form relationships and take an active role learning."

The group then created sample arguments for people who respond better to emotional appeals and for those who respond better to practical appeals. For the first type—those who are more "heart-focused"—the group said testimonials already exist from program directors and students that CBTV education leads to a better product, including increased continuity and teamwork within their programs. Also, some people may be swayed by the potential for early differentiation, which could result in more diversity in specialties and subspecialties, such as more women in surgery. The group also suggested that competency-based evaluations, which encourage relationship building, may help mitigate implicit biases held by faculty.

Finally, the group talked about improved patient care because there is, objectively, less variation in the quality of students who graduate from CBTVHPE programs.

For the second type of stakeholder—those who are more "mind-focused"—a winning argument could be that CBTVHPE is a new field of medical education research that can bring in new funding and engage junior faculty. This group also will be swayed by board scores and other outcomes measures, which currently show CBTV students to be at least equivalent to students in traditional programs. Further, the rich data that are being gathered about students in these programs will give program directors and employers more information about the capabilities of their new resident or new hire. A quick win for this group could be the fact that CBTV programs are longitudinal and learners stay in the same system, keeping known talent within the workplace and possibly attracting more support for the program from the health care system or the state.

The group also discussed what would happen if CBTVHPE were not adopted. They decided that medical education will continue to be cost prohibitive for many potential health professionals, and the system won't adapt to the needs of patients. Anticipating what naysayers might argue, the group thought some might insist that the education system isn't broken, so there is no need for CBTV education. But evidence suggests that this is wrong and that there are critical deficiencies among graduates. Other arguments might call out early differentiation as not necessarily a good thing, but the group would argue that CBTVHPE allows learners the time and space to make up their minds on a schedule that works for them. The group also raised the argument that "competency" suggests a minimum standard rather than a gold standard of excellence.

Following up on the summary of the group's discussion, one conferee mentioned research that assessed graduating residents and fellows on their abilities to perform certain procedures in a simulated environment, and they were consistently found to be "not as good as we think they are." Another conferee mentioned the results of a survey of all medical school graduates by the Association of American Medical Colleges. The survey asked graduates about their confidence levels performing the 13 core EPAs without direct supervision. The conferee mentioned several findings, but one of the most dramatic: only 54–55% of graduates said they felt confident in their abilities to enter orders and write prescriptions, even though 100% of them were doing so on the first day of residency. Another conferee summarized her own research, which found that medical students' clinical reasoning skills remain flat in the third year of medical school when they are immersed in clinical work. These and other findings mentioned by conferees support the argument that there is room for improvement in the current medical education system.

Group 5

The fifth and final group discussed ways to identify and mitigate unintended consequences of moving to a CBTVHPE model. The first and most important is ensuring that the levels of health disparities that already exist in the system don't increase. One way to mitigate this is intensive faculty development in implicit bias that then carries over into their teaching. Another type of unintended consequence could be curricular change that is undertaken as an academic exercise that doesn't actually improve outcomes—the group called this "change for change's sake." Mitigating this possibility requires rigorous outcomes research that helps identify what works and why, and the flexibility to drop components that don't work. A third possible consequence: the wasting of resources, including finances and faculty time. A robust business plan that explicitly anticipates all types of costs would help mitigate this, as well as a reward system for faculty who spend more time engaged with the educational transition.

The group also identified the need for clear and concise messaging about CBTVHPE that helps stakeholders understand what it is, how it works, and what the purpose is for doing it. Another potential consequence is a disruptive change in the culture of the health professions school. If students move through a CBTVHPE program at their own pace, they may lose their connection to their peers who are moving at their own pace. Programs will need to make adjustments so that positive aspects of the institutional culture are maintained. Related to this are the changes that faculty will experience and the need for professional development to help them adjust accordingly. The group also raised concerns about the impacts of curricular changes on partner training sites that host medical students. These external locations would need to be brought in to the planning process so that they experience minimal disruption.

Additional consequences raised by the group included the worry that CBTVHPE will produce technicians and not professionals, necessitating competencies that elevate the excellence of learners beyond a minimum set of expectations. Finally, the group reiterated the point that accreditation and regulatory bodies will need to be engaged with the concept from the beginning of any effort to introduce CBTVHPE programming. A conferee who is also an accreditor followed up on this comment by stating that accrediting bodies should be viewed as partners in driving a shift toward CBTVHPE. "We're often perceived as a barrier," she said, "but we can actually help facilitate this change."

Following the last group presentation, Drs. Lucey and Thibault wrapped up the first day of the conference by thanking the conferees and noting that the productive discussion had provided an excellent foundation for the work to come on Day 2.

DAY 2: FRIDAY, JUNE 16, 2017

Brief Recap of Day 1 and Charge to Breakout Groups

The second day of the conference began with Conference Chair Catherine Lucey reflecting on the primary themes from day one. The first theme she mentioned was the need to keep health professions education focused on patients. "Our primary goal should be moving us toward a world where peoples' health is optimized across their lifespans, regardless of what community they live in, what they look like, how they worship," she said. "I think that is an overarching agreement on the part of this group."

Another consensus point: the group agreed that the health professions can do a better job of assessing people as they move through the educational continuum. "Assessment needs to be something we think about more holistically as a path toward logical, well-paced advancement throughout a career—and it's got to be reliable," Lucey said. She explained that there are gaps in assessment that currently allow learners to progress when they're not quite ready—the group seems to agree that moving toward competency-based education is feasible and could help resolve those gaps. Related to the assessment theme is another theme: learners should be actively engaged as critical partners in their own assessment. They are "well-functioning elite learners who want to do their best and want to help optimize patient care," she said. "We're talking not about assessment **of** learning, but assessment **for** learning."

Lucey also mentioned that time variability was sometimes sidelined during the previous day's discussion, which tended to focus more heavily on competency-based education. She suggested widening the lens on time variability—defining it not just as a way to save tuition dollars and move students through programming more quickly, but viewing it as a much more expansive concept—more as individualized pacing along the continuum rather than simply program duration. The final theme from day one: that achieving competency-based, time-variable health professions education requires a clear definition, a clear value proposition, for what that looks like. "We need to ask ourselves, 'what does it look like if our systems were designed to incorporate competency-based, time-variable education? What does a practice environment look like where the physician, nurse practitioner, and pharmacist are learning optimally together and measuring that learning? We can't just make demands and expect that the leaders of our health systems and academic medical centers are going to know how to do this. We have to be part of the solution."

Dr. Lucey then handed the floor to Dr. Thibault, who provided his own summary of themes from day one. "The elements of the case we need to make on behalf of competency-based, time-variable education began to emerge yesterday," he said. "And I see two prongs to the case. One is that we need to do a better job preparing health professionals to deal with the needs of the public we serve. That is case number one—meeting the needs of patients. And two is that we have a professional responsibility to always be improving ourselves, and the CBTVHPE model helps us to fulfill that responsibility over a lifetime by facilitating continuing competency leading to professional satisfaction."

He followed up several other themes including the need for culture change within the health professions as well as the need to think more broadly about the time variability component of the model. "My concept of time variability has been expanded by the rich discussion yesterday," Thibault said. "It's as much or more about how time can be used more productively in addition to how much time is used." He also mentioned the need to accommodate different ways of implementing the model. "Not every organization is going to be able or willing to take on the level of change management that we heard described at Queen's University," he said. "There has to be accommodation for the all-in approach and also for the more gradual approach."

Following this discussion of themes, conferees then fanned out to their assigned breakout groups to continue the discussion and begin the process of developing recommendations. The five breakout groups were focused on the following topics.

- Design & Implementation of an Assessment System for CBTVHPE

- System Redesign: Curriculum Architecture, Faculty Development, and Learning Environment

- Enabling Technologies for CBTVHPE

- Continuity of Education: Managing Transitions and Learner Handoffs

- Program Evaluation: Long-Term Individual, Program, and Societal Outcomes

Plenary Session Overview: Reports from Breakout Groups, Response to Group Reports, and Identification of Missing Themes and Recommendations

Reports from Breakout Groups

After spending the morning in their breakout groups, the conferees reassembled in a plenary session to hear summary reports from each group.

Group 1: Design & Implementation of an Assessment System for CBTVHPE

This group identified several key principles to guide the design and implementation of a system of assessment within a CBTVHPE model. The first principle is embedded in the group's charge: there must be a systems-level approach to assessment, rather than "the fragmented, piecemeal efforts that we often engage in," the group's reporter said. The purpose of this systems-level approach would be to improve patient outcomes through more accurate and comprehensive assessment of learners' competencies.

The group's second principle: the assessment system must be flexible enough to meet both institutional needs and individual learner needs. It also must be longitudinal and fluid, with information able to flow through the system and not get tied up in silos. The third principle: the assessment system must be aligned with key learning and clinical outcomes. Measuring the "right" things in the best possible way ensures good decisions.

The fourth principle relates to the role of learners as co-producers in the assessment system. They should be highly activated feedback seekers within the system as well as participants in the design of the system itself, including determining how to collect, use, and share data. The fifth principle complements the fourth because it relates to the role of faculty as assessors. Faculty will also need to be involved at both levels, as assessors and users of the system and as participants in the design of the system and collection, use, and sharing of data. They also will require support and professional development as they transition into the assessor's role.

When the group's report was finished, several conferees asked about the frequency of assessment. In traditional education programs, feedback is formal and infrequent, but in competency-based programs it can occur more casually several times a day. The EPAC case study talks about learners finding frequent feedback to be more helpful and supportive of their day-to-day learning, and it can reduce their fear of negative assessments to the point that they learn to seek out feedback. A conferee also suggested that the group's guiding principles should highlight two important shifts that need to happen in the current approach to assessment— from norm-referenced to criterion-referenced assessment and from summative to formative assessment. Several other conferees made points about the need to define "systems-level assessment"—what does that look like?—and about their own breakout group's thoughts regarding a system of assessment.

Group 2: System Redesign: Curriculum Architecture, Faculty Development, and Learning Environment

This group's reporter began by describing the redesign of the learning environment: "Starting with a complete set of student learning outcomes, the learning environment is intentionally designed to create and support those outcomes," she said. "The learning environment includes the places and culture where people learn, the curriculum and its architecture, the people and their professional development." She went on to explain that, in this supportive environment, students will compete against a set of standards and not against each other with the goal of providing high-quality care to all.

In terms of the curriculum, the group stated that it would need to link all the health professions together using a shared framework with agreed upon outcomes and milestones, meaningful longitudinal experiences, and coaching for self-improvement. The group identified some key steps that would need to be taken to move toward this vision. They include 1) adopting an aligned competency-based framework across the continuum that starts with the desired outcomes in mind; 2) building a curricular nerve center composed of key stakeholders, learning experts, instructional designers to manage the curriculum and learning tools; 3) unbundling educational roles to place greater value on expertise and interprofessionalism; 4) creating continuity among interdisciplinary coaches, preceptors, clinical sites, and patients; and 5) developing a curriculum that permits flexible progression and remediation, as needed.

The group also sketched out what faculty development should look like in CBTVHPE. It should include the following: attention to diversity among faculty members, including training at all levels in implicit bias and inclusive classrooms; assessment and appropriate revision of faculty promotion and tenure guidelines; and attention to faculty skills and knowledge around new learning domains, such as social determinants of health and health systems science, and around competency-based evaluation and assessment.

Following Group 2's report, one conferee commented on the group's careful attention to interprofessional engagement and integration across the curriculum, which she said has threaded in and out of the discussions. Another commenter suggested, and many in the room agreed, that the group's vision for a CBTV curriculum should also include an interprofessional, longitudinal, integrated learning experience—not necessarily a clerkship, because that is specific to medicine, but modeled on that concept in a way that works across the health professions.

Group 3: Enabling Technologies for CBTVHPE

The third breakout group was charged with identifying the ways technology can enable or support implementation of CBTVHPE. According to its reporter, the group identified several key points. First, technology can support the concept of a learning continuum, facilitating transitions and learner handoffs and tracking learning objectives across the lifespan. Technology also can assist with the concept of longitudinal educational experiences, helping students and faculty as they follow patients over time and track learner progression over time.

Another point: technology can enhance assessment methods by making them faster, easier, more efficient, more standardized, and more robust. Technology also makes simulation possible. It also becomes a source of data over time, allowing for tracking of learners and their learning trajectories, and supports their educational planning. These same data that help individual learners also can be aggregated and analyzed to determine what works best for learners and what doesn't. And they can be used to identify and predict trends and outcomes both within and across student cohorts, departments, faculty groups, patient groups, institutions, and states, and even nationally. The group also envisioned institutions' adopting a shared technology platform across the various professions to facilitate interprofessional learning and assessment. And it discussed opportunities to create and maintain digital communities of learning within and across institutions and professions, as well as ways that technology can support individual learners and/or faculty who, for a variety of reasons, may have difficulty accessing or delivering educational programming in person. Examples might include a student in a remote area who can't afford to relocate or a retired practitioner in another city who is interested in mentoring students.

Another key point: the group acknowledged the need for committed leadership at the highest levels to ensure that an enhanced, institution-wide platform is shared, seamlessly integrated, mobile, and rapid. "Otherwise, everybody functions separately," the reporter said. In addition to high-level leadership around technology integration is the need for leadership around data stewardship. There are ethical, legal, medical, and other implications of sharing data—from learners, from faculty, from patients—that must be navigated carefully.

Following the presentation, an important conversation occurred around the need for a consortium or a similar group to help facilitate the technological shifts that institutions will need to make—in their learning management systems, their electronic health record systems, their financial aid systems, etc.—to implement CBTVHPE. "This is an expensive proposition for an institution," said one conferee. "Schools are going to have to get together to do this well."

Group 4: Continuity of Education: Managing Transitions and Learner Handoffs

Continuity of education was the focus of breakout Group 4's discussion, specifically in terms of managing transitions and learner handoffs. Like previous groups, this group also identified guiding principles, beginning with the need to define core competencies for each profession and align those competencies with the transition points in each profession. Another principle: engage accrediting, licensing, and certification bodies in enabling competency-based, time-variable learner progression, with shared accountability. This means "allowing schools to graduate learners when they are actually ready." It would also mean the development of an e-portfolio that follows health professions learners across all the transitions that they will encounter throughout their educational and professional careers.

The group also noted that time-variable transitions would require the development of flexible models for tuition, financial aid, stipends, and other administrative parts of the educational process that are currently tied to credit hours and semester units. Similarly, more flexibility would be needed in the timing of required exams, and the group recommended development of a buffer zone or a ramping up period during the transition to independent practice that would allow for continued coaching and support for recently graduated practitioners.

Another principle discussed by the group: minimizing transitions. Group members discussed creating consortia of health professions schools and institutions that would work together and share data to enable seamless transitions through a variety of arrangements. Related to this concept: the group explored standardizing the elements of transitions. This could mean, for example, a standardized approach to licensing, credentialing, and certification, such as the multi-state license concept in nursing, which reduces the testing burden on learners. The group also discussed promoting learner and trainee flexibility, enabling re-entry for those who must take time off, retraining for those who want to move into a new sphere, and compassionate off-ramps for those who leave an education or training program.

Finally, the group talked about the need to develop a supported practice model for lifelong learning. In this model, health professionals would use e-portfolios to continuously identify and track their ongoing learning goals and achievements over the course of their careers. Ideally, the model would involve coaches who work with the lifelong learners through career transitions.

Group 5: Program Evaluation: Long-Term Individual, Program, and Societal Outcomes

The final breakout group to report focused its discussion on CBTVHPE program evaluation with respect to individual, program, and societal outcomes over the long-term. The group's reporter began by suggesting that, at the societal level, CBTVHPE should be evaluated on outcomes that move society toward achieving the quadruple aim (defined as improving population health, improving the patient experience, reducing per-capita health care spending, and improving the experience of providing care for health care professionals). She then moved on to individual and program-level outcomes.

At the individual level, the group talked about CBTVHPE as an opportunity to increase alignment between internal and external assessment. This alignment would facilitate learners' believing the feedback they receive via competency-based assessment is reliable and accurate. The group also mentioned the need to develop valid assessments that allow learners to be assured that their knowledge and skill development are improving over time—that once learners have learned something, they can continue to increase their competence and that improvement can be assessed. The group also acknowledged the continuing need for remediation and also for developing admissions processes that help identify students who will succeed in CBTVHPE programs.

The group discussed improving patients' experiences and enhancing the culture of safety by training health professionals through the broad application of competency-based, time-variable education. According to the group, CBTVHPE also offers the opportunity to make health professions education more learner-centered than it is currently. It also would provide an opportunity to assess and develop the competency-based skills of faculty members who must adapt to a new educational model.

Another group member spoke about the need to determine if CBTVHPE is achieving desired outcomes as well as affecting the achievement of other health system goals, such as increasing diversity within the health professions. The speaker also mentioned the need to evaluate the implementation of all CBTVHPE programs, because schools will be transitioning to different models on varying schedules and with different challenges and resources. Using implementation science evaluation, the goal would be to identify which aspects of CBTVHPE work well, which ones do not, and which models can be more successfully implemented and/or adapted by health professions schools across the country. The speaker went on to recommend that schools that implement CBTVHPE must commit to rigorous program evaluation and be encouraged to share outcomes in a scholarly fashion to advance evidence-based educational innovations.

Response to Group Reports and Identification of Missing Themes and Recommendations

Following presentations by each of the morning breakout groups, the conferees launched into an intense discussion about what they had just heard. They were asked to focus on possible recommendations that particularly resonated with them, and to identify important points that might be missing, as well as recommendations that could be combined because they overlapped or eliminated because they were redundant or too far outside the scope of the conference.

The discussion began with Dr. Lucey asking the group to consider the role of remediation in a CBTVHPE model. Asking the group to imagine learners who, for any number of understandable reasons—such as learning differences, a personal illness or protected disability, family distractions—might take longer to master the material, she then posed the question, "To what extent can the competency-based, time-variable strategies that we've been discussing be deployed to help these students succeed, and what are the limits of our ability to use a 'mastery of learning' framework to help them?"

The first conferee to respond suggested that CBTVHPE allows educators, particularly with frequent feedback, to identify early those students who may be struggling, affording an opportunity to intervene earlier. The speaker acknowledged that, while timelines could and should be extended for students who need extra support, boundaries would need to be set around what constitutes reasonable accommodations depending on circumstances. The speaker suggested that data analytics on student performance would be helpful in navigating these circumstances.

Several other commenters followed up, some in support of retaining the language of "remediation" because it is "transparent and truthful" and others in favor of creating more "compassionate off-ramps" for students. One brought up his experience seeing fourth-year medical students dismissed from school, more likely because of problems with communication, interpersonal skills, and professionalism than for academic reasons. These areas are not currently a focus in the early years of medical school, but could be assessed earlier and more often under CBTVHPE. Conferees agreed that, regardless of what language or framework is used, CBTVHPE creates an opportunity to use data to better understand and manage the wide range of differences among students that may impact their learning timelines and educational trajectories.

The conversation then moved on to other topics, with several conferees reiterating the potential that CBTVHPE holds for faculty development and moving toward a model of continuous lifelong learning. "With all the medical and technological advances we're seeing now and will continue to see, it's important to recognize that a much more intense kind of professional development will be needed," said a conferee. "And that argues for moving toward a continuous learning model." This was something that Dr. Thibault agreed with, reiterating his belief that CBTVHPE would prepare health care professionals to fulfill their obligation for competency throughout their careers. In fact, the conferees seem to agree that an important argument to make in favor of CBTVHPE is its potential to help health professionals more explicitly fulfill their social contract with the public, to transform health care delivery for the better, and to continue to improve.

A conferee raised the need to track the trajectories of learners who go through a CBTVHPE model "because we're seeing things we haven't been able to see before, because we need to better understand more about pace and the acquisition of competencies." Another interjected that a major theme throughout the conference—that should be the focus of one or more recommendations—has been the need to invest in rigorous CBTVHPE-focused research "because there are important things we don't know."

At the same time that they seek to better understand the implications and impact of CBTVHPE, the conferees are committed to implementing at least pilot CBTVHPE programming and want to make it easier for schools to do so. "I think we should recommend aligning competencies with licensure expectations," one conferee said. "We certainly see a strong emphasis in schools of nursing on the initial licensing exam as well as graduate board scores, so aligning them does motivate behavior and influence curricular decisions." Others suggested credentialing organizations as a better fit for such a recommendation. While another cautioned conferees to think about the impact on learners because CBTVHPE—with its data gathering, coaching, and tracking—could be perceived as too intrusive a model for them. For students, the focus should be on the co-production and partnership aspects of the model—the potential for them to become more actively engaged in driving their own learning and assessment.

At this point, a conversation broke out about the onus on academic institutions to invest in this model as part of their responsibility to serve the public, to provide leadership around the research into and implementation of this model, to invest in faculty development that helps and incentivizes educators' transitions to new, unbundled roles within the model.

Drs. Lucey and Thibault then guided conferees through a discussion intended to reduce the large number of draft recommendations that had been produced by the breakout groups through prioritizing, consolidating, and eliminating. Much of this conversation focused on identifying overlaps between the recommendations of two or more groups and determining where each fit best. In some cases, a statement that began as a recommendation became a supporting argument that was relocated to the introductory essay, or preamble, that leads off the recommendations document. The group, for example, determined that the preamble should include a clear definition and vision for CBTVHPE.

"I need to take the group's temperature," said Dr. Lucey. "Before we go forward, are we ready to say that we believe competency-based, time-variable educational strategies will bring us closer to the idealized health care system that we need for our patients and populations?" The majority of the room responded affirmatively to this question. She also asked for dissenting opinions, to which one conferee said that she and several others were concerned that there is not enough evidence yet to make such a statement. Other conferees jumped in to say that the recommendations document needed to make clear that early programs are trending toward positive qualitative evidence and that ongoing research to create an evidence base for this model is a top priority. "We certainly can say that existing information, pedagogical theories, and empiric work suggest that a model such as this can make a difference, can improve on our existing model," said Lucey. "And that any institution that takes this on also takes on an obligation to study it and share results," said another conferee.

Another commenter said, "I think we can say something along the lines of this: we don't believe that the current system, which is a 100-year-old relic, is adequately preparing folks, and we believe that CBTVHPE aligns with the learning science and the needs of patients and the current health care system, and should be pursued—gathering data in the process for more widespread implementation—to fulfill our contract with society."

Dr. Lucey then called again for anyone with concerns or hesitations to speak up, and one conferee did—raising concerns about her own institution's capacity to take on a transition to CBTVHPE at this time. "I just can't imagine, particularly at this moment in time with the budgetary challenges we're facing and all the other realities, that this would go well," she said. "Even though we do have faculty who would definitely want to try this and, without institutional commitment and leadership, it would not go well."

The conferee was thanked for her candor and the group agreed that there would need to be messaging in the recommendations around the diffusion of innovation. The document must acknowledge that not all schools—particularly smaller schools not affiliated with an academic health center and those more dependent on tuition dollars—will be able to pursue this fully or even partially, if at all, at this time. All schools, however, will learn valuable information, such as best practices, from the early adopters of CBTVHPE, and sharing that information widely will be critically important going forward.

At the close of day two, committee members worked on drafting recommendations from the breakout groups that they had facilitated and/or participated in, while Dr. Lucey and Macy staff worked on the introduction and conference overview sections. Overnight, these different sections were combined into one complete first draft and distributed to the conferees for review.

DAY 3: SATURDAY, JUNE 17, 2017

On day three, the conferees came together to share their feedback on the draft recommendations document.

Conference Conclusions and Recommendations

Conferees were generous with their praise and also shared many substantive comments intended to strengthen the first draft of the recommendations document. Many, for example, felt that the opening paragraphs lacked "oomph" and failed to create a "burning platform" to draw in readers. This dovetailed with a discussion about the need to provide more background and context regarding the challenges facing America's health care system. Overall, the conferees felt strongly that the introduction needed to convey more provocatively the imperative for pursuing CBTVHPE.

One conferee stated, for example, that, "There isn't anything in there about how we're worried that we're graduating individuals who aren't perfectly confident or competent or about the massive environmental changes happening that would create a call to action."

Constructive criticism about the opening paragraphs led to a discussion about tone, with conferees expressing concerns about the occasionally negative tone of the introduction. Several conferees thought that, while the paper must convey the overwhelming nature of the rapidly evolving challenges facing the health system, it should frame the current situation as an opportunity to improve a system that has always strived for and often achieved excellence.

On another topic, some conferees expressed or agreed that the draft seemed too "physician-centric"—too focused around medical education and practice—and not inclusive enough of other the health professions. "We should be more purposeful about using language that cuts across all health professions," a conferee said. Along the same vein, others felt that it did not adequately characterize the potential interprofessional benefits of CBTVHPE.

Regarding overall content and organization of the document, conferees debated the optimal grouping and ordering of the recommendations, worked on winnowing the total number of recommendations, and wrestled with the specificity of the recommendations, discussing how prescriptive versus suggestive to be and how to create consistency across recommendations. At Dr. Thibault's invitation, the conferees agreed to think about and forward to the writing committee draft suggestions for a consensus vision statement about CBTVHPE to be included in the introduction. "We often include in these Macy recommendations reports a vision statement that defines for our readers what it is we want to achieve with our recommendations," he said.

The conversation continued throughout the morning, moving from overarching comments about style, tone, and organization to more granular suggestions regarding specific recommendations and sections that required additional work. During this part of the discussion, the conferees called for more consistency in the language used, fewer assumptions about what the audience may already know, clearer definitions of certain concepts, the insertion of examples to support important points, and much more. Often, during this part of the conversation, conferees would identify important points that first appeared only in the recommendations, but that needed to be stated more explicitly in the preamble first. For example, while talking about recommendations related to research and faculty development, the conferees realized that both these topics needed a stronger foundation in the introduction.

Upon conclusion of the discussion, the writing committee was charged with revising the draft recommendations document based on the feedback provided by the conferees. In the weeks following the conference, the committee revised and reviewed numerous versions of the draft via email and phone meetings, with two iterations, including a semi-final draft, distributed to all conferees for review and comment. The final, consensus document appears in this monograph.

Drs. Thibault and Lucey then formally closed the conference by thanking the planning/writing committee, the participants, and the Macy Foundation staff. Dr. Thibault said, "At this point in the meeting, we're all exhausted, but there's a sense of exhilaration and accomplishment, and I want to thank you all for what you've given to us here, for participating fully. Isn't it wonderful that we have important work to do and wonderful people to do it with?"

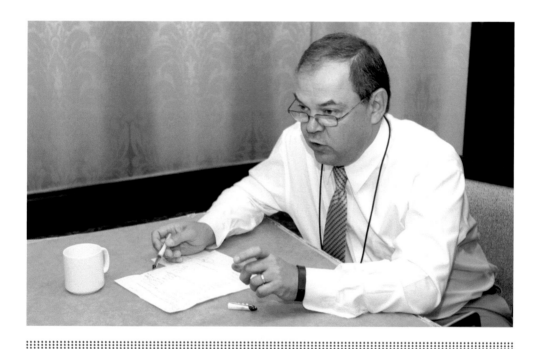

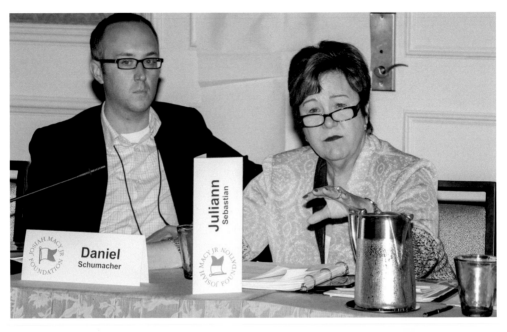

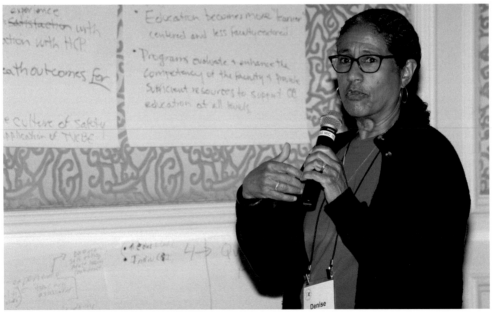

SELECTED BIBLIOGRAPHY

Required

1. Schuwirth L, Ash J. Assessing tomorrow's learners: In competency-based education only a radically different holistic method of assessment will work. Six things we could forget. *Med Teach*. 2013;35:555–559. doi: 10.3109/0142159X.2013.787140.

2. Carraccio C, Englander R, Holmboe ES, Kogan JR. Driving care quality: Aligning trainee assessment and supervision through practical application of entrustable professional activities, competencies, and milestones. *Acad Med*. 2016;91(2):199–203. doi: 10.1097/ACM.0000000000000985.

3. Holmboe ES, Foster TC, Ogrinc G. Co-creating quality in health care through learning and dissemination. *J Contin Educ Health Prof*. 2016;36(1):S16–S18. doi: 10.1097/CEH.0000000000000076.

Supplemental

1. Eva KW, Bordage G, Campbell C, et al. Towards a program of assessment for health professionals: From training into practice. *Adv Health Sci Educ Theory Pract* 2016;21:897–913. doi 10.1007/s10459-015-9653-6.

2. Garrett R, Lurie H. Deconstructing competency-based education: An assessment of institutional activity, goals, and challenges in higher education. Boston, MA: Ellucian: 2016.

3. Tavares W, Ginsburg S, Eva K. Selecting & simplifying: Rater performance and behavior when considering multiple competencies. *Teach Learn Med*. 2016;28(1):41–51. DOI: 10.1080/10401334.2015.1107489.

4. Kelchen R. The landscape of competency-based education: Enrollments, demographics, and affordability. Washington, DC: Center on Higher Education Reform, American Enterprise Institute: 2015.

5. Holmboe E, Batalden P. Achieving the desired transformation: Thoughts on next steps for outcomes-based medical education *Acad Med.* 2015;90(9):1215–1223. doi: 10.1097/ACM.0000000000000779.

6. Norman G, Norcini J, Bordage G. Competency-based education: Milestones or millstones. *J Grad Med Educ.* 2014;6(1):1–6. doi: http://dx.doi.org/10.4300/JGME-D-13-00445.1.

7. Albanese M, Mejicano G, Mullan P, Kokotailo P, Gruppen L. Defining characteristics of educational competencies. *Med Educ.* 2008;42:248–255. doi:10.1111/j.1365-2923.2007.02996.x.

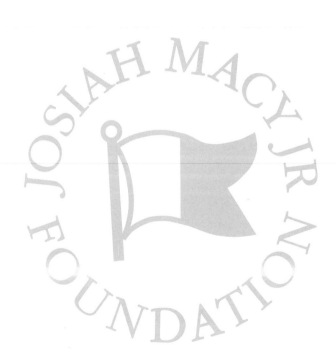

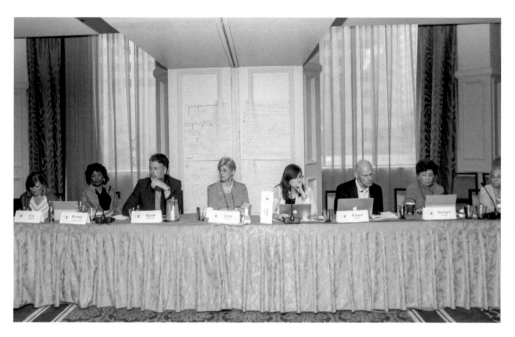

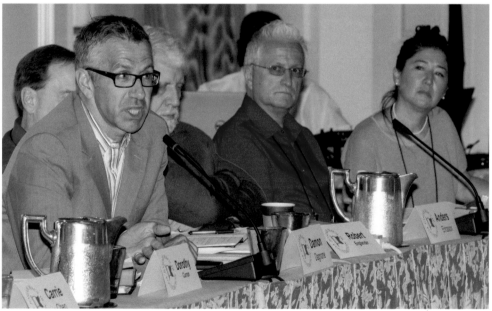

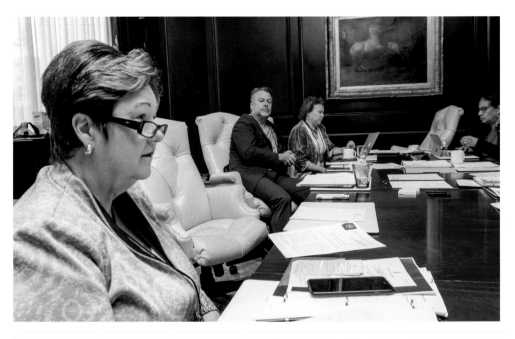

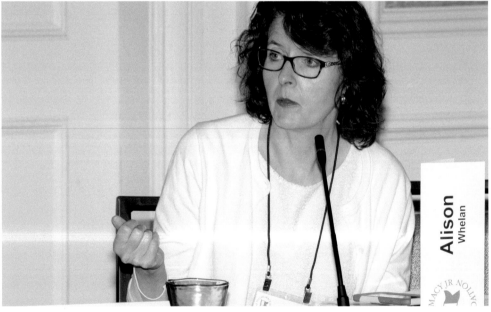

BIOGRAPHIES
OF PARTICIPANTS

Eva Aagaard, MD, FACP

Eva Aagaard, MD, FACP, is Professor of Medicine and Senior Associate Dean for Education at Washington University School of Medicine. In these roles, she oversees medical education across the continuum including undergraduate (UME), graduate (GME) and continuing medical education. At University of Colorado School of Medicine, she developed and served as Founding Director of their internationally recognized Academy of Medical Educators. Nationally she led development of the Society of General Internal Medicine TEACH Program. Internationally she developed the Health Education Advanced Leadership Program in Zimbabwe (HEALZ). Dr. Aagaard is a member of the American Board of Internal Medicine Specialty Board, Council Member for the Society of General Internal Medicine, and past co-chair of the National Board of Medical Examiners Ambulatory Care Test Development Committee and several item review committees. She served as a core member of the Milestones in Internal Medicine Committee. Her areas of interest include curriculum reform, competency-based education, and assessment and teaching across the continuum of health professions education from UME through practicing provider. She has won more than 15 awards for clinical excellence, teaching, and humanism in medicine, including the University of Colorado's President's Teaching Award, the Society of General Internal Medicine Mid-Career Mentoring Award, and the Elizabeth Gee Award for the Advancement of Women at the University of Colorado.

G. Rumay Alexander, EdD, MSN, BSN, FAAN

G. Rumay Alexander, EdD, MSN, BSN, FAAN, is Professor and Director of the Office of Inclusive Excellence at The University of North Carolina at Chapel Hill School of Nursing; and Associate Vice Chancellor and Chief Diversity Officer of the university. She has a compelling record of leadership and advocacy for diversity and inclusive excellence in academia, the workplace, in national nursing professional organizations, and in her consultant activities. She provides leadership not only for the school of nursing but also for the Gilling's School of Global Public Health, the UNC School of Dentistry, and UNC's Faculty Governance's Community and Diversity Committee. Her passion centers on intentional efforts to resource the proper understanding and judicious application of equity and multicultural concepts for students, faculty, personnel and the patients served by UNC health professions graduates. These efforts include the facilitation of system-wide efforts to give respect to the many dimensions of human difference as well as the lived experience of difference.

Dr. Alexander is known for helping organizations succeed in their missions. Her participation in high impact initiatives, numerous consultations and presentations nationally and internationally, and professional organization work devoted to generational equity bear witness to her game-changing works. She has guided individuals in academic, corporate, health care, and religious organizations to explore marginalizing processes, multiple perspectives, and the vicissitudes of lived experiences of difference, and has authored numerous articles, books, and book chapters. Her passion for equity of opportunity and penchant for holding courageous dialogues to steward and promote human flourishing has led to appointments on landmark health care initiatives, including the Commission of Workforce for Hospitals and Health Systems of the American Hospital Association and the National Quality Forum's steering committee for the first national voluntary consensus standards for nursing-sensitive care. She is a two-term member on the Board of Governors of the National League for Nursing and the American Organization of Nurse Executives. In 2010, she was the recipient of the American Organization of Nurse Executive's Prism Award for workforce diversity leadership and in 2013, the National Student Nurses' Association bestowed her with their most prestigious award of Honorary Membership. In addition, she received the Southern Regional Education Board's M. Elizabeth Carnegie Award in 2013.

Dr. Alexander holds a baccalaureate degree in nursing from the University of Tennessee Knoxville, a master's degree in nursing from Vanderbilt University, and a doctor of education degree from Tennessee State University.

David L. Battinelli, MD

David L. Battinelli, MD, is Dean for Medical Education and the Betsy Cushing Whitney Professor of Medicine at the Hofstra Northwell School of Medicine. Dr. Battinelli is responsible for the overall professional management of clinical, educational, research and operational issues related to medical and clinical affairs. Previously, he served as the health system's chief academic officer and senior vice president of academic affairs, in charge of all undergraduate and graduate educational programs, all continuing medical education, and academic affairs and institutional relationships.

A board-certified internist, Dr. Battinelli came to Northwell Health (formerly the North Shore-LIJ Health System) from Boston Medical Center (BMC) where he served as vice chairman for education; program director, internal medicine residency program; and professor of medicine at Boston University School of Medicine. He was also an active staff physician at BMC and the Boston Veterans Administration.

Dr. Battinelli is a past-president of the Association of Program Directors in Internal Medicine. He has worked closely with and served on numerous committees for a variety of national medical organizations, including the Alliance for Academic Internal Medicine, American Board of Internal Medicine, American College of Physicians, and the Accreditation Committee on Graduate Medical Education, among others. In addition, he has lectured extensively on clinical education, faculty development of teaching skills and internal medicine, and is a noted workshop leader and author on these subjects.

Dr. Battinelli earned his medical degree from the University of Medicine and Dentistry, Newark, NJ, and a Bachelor of Science degree from the University of Scranton, Scranton, PA.

Anne Bavier, PhD, RN, FAAN

Anne Bavier, PhD, RN, FAAN, Dean of the College of Nursing and Health Innovation, oversees the largest academic unit at the University of Texas at Arlington.

Approximately 40 percent of the university's 54,000 students are enrolled in the College of Nursing and Health Innovation. The college is the largest producer of registered nurses in the state of Texas and one of the five largest nursing programs in the United States.

A leading voice on health care, Dr. Bavier is the president of the National League for Nursing, an organization of nearly 40,000 faculty nurses and leaders in nursing education. She received the Gold Medallion from the Chapel of the Four Chaplains, a rare honor for a civilian and only the second nurse so honored, for her dedicated service to the nation.

She is a former senior official of the National Institutes of Health and has served as nursing dean of two top-ranked institutions: the University of Connecticut and Saint Xavier University. Since signing on as dean in 2014, Dr. Bavier has led the College of Nursing and Health Innovation through a remarkable transformation, including a merger with the Department of Kinesiology and the recruitment of several internationally renowned health care scholars and researchers who are making significant contributions to improving health and the human condition.

Under Bavier's leadership, the college was designated a National League for Nursing Center for Excellence, making it one of only a dozen colleges of nursing in the country that has been so honored.

She is a sought-after speaker, on topics ranging from academic leadership to health care policy and innovation. Her speaking engagements include international organizations, such as Universitas 21 and Oxford Round Table. Her editorials in newspapers and health business journals are cited for their breadth and depth of understanding of the pressures facing health care systems and providers.

Dr. Bavier holds an undergraduate degree in nursing from Duke, a master of nursing from Emory and a doctoral degree from Duquesne.

Lisa M. Bellini, MD

Lisa M. Bellini, MD, obtained her medical degree from the University of Alabama in 1990. She came to Penn to pursue her Internal Medicine residency training followed by a year as Chief Medical Resident. She subsequently completed a Pulmonary Fellowship and joined the faculty in 1996.

Dr. Bellini currently serves as Vice Chair of Education for the Department of Medicine. In that role, she is responsible for education in the Department of Medicine. As Program Director of the Internal Medicine Residency since 1996, she directly oversees 154 residents in one of the nation's best training programs and is indirectly responsible for the training of an additional 150 subspecialty fellows.

From 2005–2008, she was Associate Dean for Graduate Medical Education and Designated Institutional Official for University of Pennsylvania Health System. In that role, she had operational responsibility for all policies and procedures related to the training of residents and fellows in all 68 UPHS-sponsored training programs as well as ensured that all programs were operating in substantial compliance with the ACGME institutional and program requirements.

From 2008–2016, she was Vice Dean for Faculty Affairs for the Perelman School of Medicine. In that role, she had oversight of faculty policies and procedures in the Perelman School of Medicine at the University Pennsylvania. In 2016, she assumed the role of Vice Dean for Academic Affairs for the Perelman School of Medicine.

On a national level, Dr. Bellini is an active member of the Alliance of Academic Internal Medicine (AAIM) where she served as inaugural Chair of the Board. AAIM is a consortium of five academically focused specialty organizations representing departments of internal medicine at medical schools and teaching hospitals in the United States and Canada. It represents department chairs and chiefs; clerkship, residency, and fellowship program directors; division chiefs; and academic and business administrators as well as other faculty and staff in departments of internal medicine and their divisions. Previously, she has held the positions of Treasurer and President of the Association for Program Directors in Internal Medicine. She has also served on several key committees for the Accreditation Council for Graduate Medical Education, using much of her research and administrative experience to influence national policy regarding graduate medical education. She was also a member of the Institute of Medicine's committee on Conflict of Interest, which has had a major impact on professional conduct within the academic community.

Her research focuses on medical education, including the health and well-being of residents and faculty as well as the effects of fatigue and sleep deprivation on patient outcomes and the learning environment.

Robert (Bob) A. Blouin, PharmD

Robert A. "Bob" Blouin is Executive Vice Chancellor and Provost ("provost") of The University of North Carolina at Chapel Hill. The provost serves as the chief operating officer of the university and works in unison with the chancellor to lead critically important pan-university initiatives. The provost also has oversight responsibilities for budget and planning.

Alongside Chancellor Carol Folt, Blouin plays a central leadership role in implementing Carolina's first-ever strategic framework, an initiative that will guide university growth over the next decade. He believes a key mission of the provost is to ensure Carolina attracts, develops, and retains leading faculty members focused on preparing students for success in a rapidly changing global economy.

An acclaimed educator, award-winning researcher, and internationally recognized innovator, Blouin was Dean of the UNC Eshelman School of Pharmacy from 2003 to 2017. When announcing Blouin as Carolina's 15th Provost, Chancellor Folt cited his exceptional professionalism as dean and his change-leadership success that has helped accelerate the school's unprecedented expansion and international recognition in its research, education, and global engagement programs. He will continue to serve as the school's Bryson Distinguished Professor.

During his tenure as dean, the UNC Eshelman School of Pharmacy was recognized as one of the premier pharmacy programs in the world as evidenced by its rankings with US News & World Reports, QS World University Rankings in Pharmacy and Pharmacology and AACP grants and contracts. In addition, the school initiated a first-of-its-kind professional degree granting partnership program in Asheville, North Carolina, which focuses on ambulatory care and rural health. Under Blouin's leadership, the faculty research portfolio increased from $2 million in 2002 to $36 million in 2016, ranking second among the nation's pharmacy schools. As director of the Eshelman Institute for Innovation, Blouin also led a cutting-edge effort to find creative ways to accelerate change in education and health care.

Blouin is noted for his leadership of national discussions on issues of clinical pharmaceutical scientist training, particularly at the graduate level. He has been extensively involved in launching a transformation in the professional and graduate curricula at Carolina coined the Educational Renaissance. His own research interests include studying the effect of disease and altered physiologic status on the pharmacokinetics, pharmacodynamics, and metabolism of drugs.

Before coming to Carolina, Blouin was a faculty member and administrator at the University of Kentucky College of Pharmacy from 1978 to 2003. There, he took on the role of associate dean for research and graduate education in 1997, where his responsibilities included overseeing the development and expansion of the Center for Pharmaceutical Sciences and Technology. Additionally, as the executive director of the Office for Economic Development and Innovations Management, he served as the College of Pharmacy representative on all issues external to the University of Kentucky and those relating to economic development of the pharmaceutical sciences. He also represented the college on several statewide biotechnology initiatives and has worked to advance faculty-based intellectual property.

A native of Massachusetts, Blouin earned a BS from the Massachusetts College of Pharmacy and a PharmD from the University of Kentucky College of Pharmacy. He lives in Chapel Hill with his wife, Maureen. They have a daughter, a son, and three granddaughters.

Barbara F. Brandt, PhD

Barbara F. Brandt, PhD, is renowned for her work in health professional education, and specifically, interprofessional education and continuing education. Dr. Brandt serves as the associate vice president for education within the University of Minnesota's Academic Health Center, and she is responsible for the University's *1Health* initiative to build the interprofessional practice skills of students and faculty in a broad range of health professions. Dr. Brandt is also the director of the National Center for Interprofessional Practice and Education, a public-private partnership and cooperative agreement with the Health Resources and Services Administration, established in 2012.

In her leadership roles, Dr. Brandt has served as a consultant, advisor and speaker for a wide variety of organizations such as the Institute of Medicine, the National Quality Forum, the Academy of Healthcare Improvement, the Josiah Macy Jr. Foundation, the Association of Schools of Allied Health Professions, the American Speech-Language-Hearing Association, and the American Medical Association.

Dr. Brandt holds a bachelor of arts in the teaching of history from the University of Illinois at Chicago and a master of education and doctor of philosophy degrees in continuing education (specializing in continuing professional education for the health professions) from the University of Illinois at Urbana-Champaign. In 2013, she was recognized as a University of Illinois Distinguished Alumna. She completed a W.K. Kellogg Foundation-sponsored post-doctoral fellowship for faculty in adult and continuing education at the University of Wisconsin-Madison.

Aaron Brower, PhD

Aaron Brower, PhD, is Provost and Vice Chancellor of University of Wisconsin (UW)-Extension, a position he began in 2012 and resumed after serving as Interim Chancellor of UW Colleges and UW-Extension in 2014.

As Provost and Vice Chancellor, Brower provides strategic and operational leadership as UW-Extension's chief academic officer. He oversees its four major divisions (Continuing Education and Online Learning, Public Radio and Television, Business and Entrepreneurship, and Cooperative Extension); provides administrative support for business and finance; and develops and supports collaborative programs between UW-Extension and all 26 institutions within the University of Wisconsin System.

Brower helped create, and continues to lead, the UW Flexible Option (UW Flex), the competency-based educational program for the UW System and State of Wisconsin. UW Flex is the first-in-the-country program that provides students a way to receive degrees and certificates through competency-based and direct-assessment methods from existing public higher education institutions.

Prior to joining UW-Extension, Brower was UW-Madison's Vice Provost for Teaching & Learning, where he was responsible for guiding and supporting undergraduate education and professional development. Brower remains a tenured professor at UW-Madison in the School of Social Work, and in the departments of Integrated Liberal Studies and Educational Leadership & Policy Analysis. He was the principal investigator for over $18 million in grants, and has written more than 50 articles on student learning, student life, and student success.

Brower's expertise is in educational innovations, project-based learning, student learning and outcome assessment, engaging the whole university on issues important to students and the people of Wisconsin. His work demonstrates that students' academic and social outcomes are produced when college environments blend in- and out-of-class learning and experiences to create communities of students, faculty, and staff who share common learning goals (i.e., learning communities). He has created and led many teaching and learning programs focused on integrative learning and evidence-based curricular reform, with an emphasis on high-impact learning practices.

Brower earned his BA in psychology, MSW, MA in psychology, and PhD in social work and psychology from the University of Michigan. He is the recipient of several awards for his work, including being named in 2006 as one of the nation's *Outstanding First-Year Student Advocates* by Houghton Mifflin and the National Resource Center for the First-Year Experience.

Carol Carraccio, MD, MA

Carol Carraccio, MD, MA, is a general pediatrician, who completed her residency training at St. Christopher's Hospital for Children in Philadelphia and her Robert Wood Johnson fellowship in general academic pediatrics at the Children's Hospital of Philadelphia. She spent the first 25 years of her career as a residency program director at the University of Maryland. At the time that competency-based medical education was introduced, she went back to Loyola College to earn her master's degree in education. During these years, she also became Associate Chair for Education and a tenured Professor of Pediatrics. Dr. Carraccio took on many national leadership roles, including the Milestone Project for the pediatrics community, President of the Association of Pediatric Program Directors, Chair of the Accreditation Council for Graduate Medical Education Review Committee for Pediatrics, and Director of the Initiative for Innovation in Pediatric Education. In 2011, she was recruited by The American Board of Pediatrics to become the Vice-President of Competency-Based Assessment. Her current work focuses on the integration of competencies/milestones with entrustable professional activities (EPAs) as a practical framework for learner assessment across the continuum of education, training, and practice. She is involved in several research projects that are introducing EPAs into learner assessment, including Education in Pediatrics Across the Continuum (EPAC), an AAMC initiative that has received support from the Josiah Macy Jr. Foundation.

Kathy Chappell, PhD, RN, FNAP, FAAN

Kathy Chappell, PhD, RN, FNAP, FAAN, is Senior Vice President of Certification, Measurement, Accreditation and Research at the American Nurses Credentialing Center. She is responsible for certification of individual registered nurses and advanced practice registered nurses and for development of certification examinations. She is responsible for the accreditation of organizations that provide continuing nursing education and interprofessional continuing education, and for accreditation of residency and fellowship programs for nurses. She also directs the Institute for Credentialing Research, analyzing outcomes related to credentialing.

She holds a baccalaureate in nursing with distinction from the University of Virginia, a master of science in advanced clinical nursing and a doctorate in nursing from George Mason University. She is a Fellow in the American Academy of Nursing and a Distinguished Scholar & Fellow in the National Academies of Practice.

H. Carrie Chen, MD, PhD

H. Carrie Chen, MD, PhD, is Associate Dean of Assessment and Educational Scholarship and Professor of Pediatrics at Georgetown University School of Medicine. She previously held a faculty appointment at University of California, San Francisco (UCSF) for several years where she was a member of the Academy of Medical Educators, held the Abraham Rudolph Endowed Chair in Pediatric Education, and continues to consult on Education in Pediatrics Across the Continuum (EPAC), an AAMC-sponsored competency-based education pilot in pediatrics. She has robust experience with pre-clerkship, clerkship, fourth-year medical student, residency, fellowship, and continuing medical education as well as faculty development. These experiences include curricular design; program development, implementation, and leadership; and educational research. She recently received her PhD in Health Professions Education and completed a visiting professorship at the Center for Research and Development of Education at the University Medical Center Utrecht in the Netherlands. Her research interests include student engagement for workplace learning, workplace-based assessments, including the use of entrustable professional activities, and faculty skill development and support.

Dorothy Curran, MD

Dorothy Curran, MD, is a first-year Pediatric Resident at the University of Minnesota, and is part of the first cohort in the AAMC initiative Education in Pediatrics Across the Continuum (EPAC). She has participated in local and national meetings shaping the EPAC program, which tests the feasibility of medical education and training that is based on the demonstration of defined outcomes rather than on time, from early in medical school through completion of residency.

She is currently working on a scholarly project on the Sub-Internship experience for EPAC, and is very interested in exploring ways to promote a culture of feedback in both undergraduate and graduate medicine that is focused, timely, and less intimidating for both supervisors and trainees.

Dorothy graduated from the Massachusetts Institute of Technology and the University of Minnesota Medical School. She has research interests and projects in community participatory research, health care disparities, pediatric emergency medicine, and pediatric cancer survivorship.

J. Damon Dagnone, MD, FRCPC, MSc, MMEd

J. Damon Dagnone, MD, FRCPC, MSc, MMEd, is Associate Professor of Emergency Medicine and the competency-based medical education (CBME) Faculty Lead for Postgraduate Medical Education at Queen's University. His previous research has focused on simulation-based curriculum development, OSCE assessment, and other innovative teaching and learning methods. Over the last seven years, Dr. Dagnone has also been the director of both university and national resuscitation competitions in simulation held annually. Currently, he is immersed in helping develop a national framework for high-stakes, simulation-based OSCE assessment in resuscitation, and is working towards developing a clinical resuscitation assessment tool for trainees. As the CBME faculty lead, and Special Assistant to the Associate Dean of Postgraduate Medical Education, Dr. Dagnone has become immersed in numerous institutional and collaborative research projects which include competency-based curricular methods, assessment frameworks, program evaluation, and conceptual papers, both within the university and in partnership with the Royal College of Physicians and Surgeons of Canada. Stay tuned for an exciting next few years in his research career.

Please feel free to contact Dr. Dagnone (jdd1@queensu.ca) at any time regarding his research interests and expertise in simulation-based medical education and the evolving realm of research within CBME.

Robert Englander, MD, MPH

Robert Englander, MD, MPH, recently moved to Minneapolis to assume the role of Associate Dean for Undergraduate Medical Education at the University of Minnesota Medical School. He received his MD degree from Yale in 1987 and an MPH from Johns Hopkins in 1999. Bob completed a Pediatrics residency at the Children's National Medical Center in Washington, DC, and a fellowship in Pediatric Critical Care Medicine at the Massachusetts General Hospital in Boston. From 1993–2002, Bob was at the University of Maryland as a Pediatric Intensivist, where his roles included Associate Director of the Residency Training Program in Pediatrics and Director of Undergraduate Medical Studies for the Department of

Pediatrics. In 2002, Bob relocated to Hartford, Connecticut, to be Medical Director of Inpatient Services and to start an academic division of hospital medicine at the Connecticut Children's Medical Center and the University of Connecticut School of Medicine. From 2005–2011, he assumed the role of Vice President and then Senior Vice President for Quality and Patient Safety. During his years in Connecticut, Bob also served as Associate Director of the Pediatric Residency Training Program, overseeing competency-based education; served on the Board of Directors of the Association of Pediatric Program Directors; and was a member of the Pediatrics Milestones Working Group.

In 2011, Bob moved to the AAMC, where his efforts were aimed at advancing competency-based medical education. He served as the project lead for Education in Pediatrics Across the Continuum (EPAC), a model that seeks to advance students from medical school through residency based on competence rather than time. Bob also served as the AAMC's project lead and one of the drafting panel members for the recent publication of the Core Entrustable Professional Activities for Entering Residency. Bob left the AAMC in May 2015 and was an Adjunct Professor of Pediatrics at the George Washington University School of Medicine and a consultant to The American Board of Pediatrics on alternate pathways for Maintenance of Certification Part IV and the development of Entrustable Professional Activities for the specialty of Pediatrics.

K. Anders Ericsson, PhD

K. Anders Ericsson, PhD, is presently Conradi Eminent Scholar and Professor of Psychology at Florida State University. After completing his PhD in Sweden, he collaborated with the Nobel Prize winner in Economics Herbert A. Simon on verbal reports of thinking, leading to their classic book *Protocol Analysis: Verbal Reports as Data* (1984). Currently he studies the measurement of expert performance in domains such as music, chess, nursing, law enforcement, and sports, and how expert performers attain their superior performance by acquiring complex cognitive mechanisms and physiological adaptations through extended deliberate practice. He has edited the *Cambridge Handbook of Expertise and Expert Performance* which will come out in a second edition this fall. His most recent book (2016) *Peak: Secrets from the new science of expertise* was co-authored with Robert Pool. He has published articles in prestigious journals, such as *Science, Psychological Review, Psychological Bulletin, Current Biology,* and *Trends of Cognitive Science.* He is a Fellow of the Center for Advanced Study in the Behavioral Sciences, of the American Psychological Association and the Association for Psychological Science, and a member of the

Royal Swedish Academy of Engineering Sciences. His research has been featured in cover stories in *Scientific American*, *Time*, *Fortune*, the *Wall Street Journal*, and the *New York Times*. He has been invited to give keynote presentations at conferences of surgeons, musicians, teachers, clinical psychologists, athletes, and coaches as well as professional sports organizations, such as the Philadelphia Eagles (American football), San Antonio Spurs (basketball), and Manchester City (soccer).

Jeffrey J. Evans, PhD

Jeffrey J. Evans, PhD, studied music performance, focusing on trumpet and flugelhorn, and sharing the stage with legends in the entertainment industry prior to earning his BS from Purdue. Engaging in two simultaneous careers as a musician and practicing electrical engineer, he toured the United States and Europe, and released a CD of his original compositions, gaining critical acclaim in the US, South America, and Europe. As an electrical engineer, he designed products in medical diagnostics, automotive powertrain control, telecommunications, and consumer safety. His products have sold tens of millions, and saved thousands of lives. During the later stages of his 22 years in industry, he "re-tooled," earning his MS and PhD degrees in Computer Science from the Illinois Institute of Technology, focusing on communications network performance and adaptive systems on distributed systems such as clusters, Grids, and sensor networks. During this time, he was heavily involved with systems and software design of Hybrid Fiber-Coax infrastructure in the telecommunications industry.

Dr. Evans works to understand the mechanisms that disrupt complex systems. His research has included the impact of communication performance degradation on parallel application run time. He has applied his research in adaptive computing systems to the areas of sensor networks in hydrologic applications and human physical activity monitoring. His explorations also include performance management of large-scale distributed hardware-in-the-loop simulations of vehicles, molecular dynamics simulations of nano-scale machining operations used in manufacturing, and molecular dynamics simulations of fire events. Recently Dr. Evans has been investigating hardware-in-the-loop simulations of data networks used in real-time applications related to audio and video delivery in live performance situations. He is currently investigating the use of artificial intelligence for use in live music composition and performance.

Since 2013, Dr. Evans has dedicated himself to transforming higher education as a founding faculty fellow in the Polytechnic incubator. He has co-developed largely lecture-less learning experiences that cross-cut and balance STEM fields and the humanities for the purpose of developing learner cognitive and meta-cognitive competencies needed for lifelong success in the 21st century. In 2015, he spearheaded the architecture and development of an innovative competency-based undergraduate program called Transdisciplinary Studies in Technology, the first of its kind at a major R1 university. The program has been approved by Purdue University and the state of Indiana, who called the program a "game changer," and was approved by Purdue's regional accrediting body in March 2016.

Tonya L. Fancher, MD, MPH

Tonya L. Fancher, MD, MPH, is Associate Dean of Workforce Innovation and Community Engagement at the University of California Davis (UC Davis) School of Medicine. A primary care-trained general internist, Dr. Fancher spent four years in the US Air Force and then completed her MPH and Health Services Research Fellowship at UC Davis. For the past ten years, she has led undergraduate and graduate medical education Title VII grants focused on bolstering the primary care workforce in vulnerable communities. She is currently the Director of the HRSA-supported Center for a Diverse Healthcare Workforce and the PI on an American Medical Association grant for a six-year accelerated primary care pathway linking medical school to primary care GME programs at UC Davis and Kaiser Permanente Northern California.

Nelda Godfrey, PhD, ACNS-BC, RN, FAAN

Nelda Godfrey, PhD, ACNS-BC, RN, FAAN, is Professor and Associate Dean of Innovative Partnerships and Practice at the University of Kansas School of Nursing. She led the KU undergraduate faculty as Associate Dean for Undergraduate Programs as faculty designed and implemented a concept-based curriculum, and has led interprofessional educational efforts at the academic health center since 2008. Situated on a medical center campus with a school of nursing, school of medicine, and a school of health professions, Dr. Godfrey was also part of the research team that found that outcomes in the category of professional identity and communication constituted one-fourth of the *AACN Baccalaureate Essentials for Professional Nursing Practice* (2008) identified outcomes. She has developed and taught the BSN program's Introduction to the Profession course, the first in a series of three professional development courses in the BSN curriculum. A recognized scholar in professional identity formation and nursing education transformation,

Dr. Godfrey now leads in the School of Nursing as Associate Dean for Innovative Partnerships and Practice.

Dr. Godfrey has a BSN from the University of Missouri, a master's degree with Clinical Nurse Specialist preparation from the University of Kansas, and a PhD in Nursing from the University of Missouri. She serves as the chair of the Standards Committee for the National League for Nursing Commission on Nursing Education Accreditation, and as a member of the American Nurses Association Ethics and Human Rights Advisory Board. Dr. Godfrey and her husband live in Liberty, Missouri.

Larry D. Gruppen, PhD

Larry D. Gruppen, PhD, is Professor in the Department of Learning Health Sciences at the University of Michigan Medical School, where he directs the competency-based Master in Health Professions Education program. His research interests center around the development of expertise, knowledge and performance assessment, self-regulated learning, and educational leadership development. He has held the offices of president of the Society of Directors of Research in Medical Education and chair of the Association of American Medical College's (AAMC) Central Group on Educational Affairs. He was also the founding Chair of the AAMC's Medical Education Research Certificate (MERC) program. He has over 140 peer-reviewed publications on a variety of topics in medical education and presents regularly at national and international professional meetings. He was recognized for career productivity by the AAMC's Central Group for Educational Affairs' Medical Education Laureate Award, the 2015 John P. Hubbard Award from the National Board of Medical Examiners, and the Merrel Flair Award from the AAMC Group on Educational Affairs.

Richard E. Hawkins, MD, FACP

Richard E. Hawkins, MD, FACP, joined the American Medical Association (AMA) in December 2012 as Vice President for Medical Education Programs. He is responsible for providing senior staff leadership and support to the AMA's Council on Medical Education and Academic Physician Section. He also provides staff leadership for the AMA's Accelerating Change in Education project, a broad initiative designed to better prepare medical school graduates to practice and learn in an evolving health care environment. Dr. Hawkins has more than 20 years of experience working on various initiatives to evaluate and improve physician performance, and is co-editor of a textbook on the assessment of clinical competence. Prior to joining the AMA, Dr. Hawkins was senior vice president for professional and scientific affairs at the American Board of Medical Specialties (ABMS). At ABMS, he worked with staff, committees, and external stakeholders to help promote the science of ABMS Maintenance of Certification® and certification in the context of advancing physician assessment programs. He also led in the formation of ABMS-International and development of its certification and examination programs. Prior to assuming his position with ABMS, Dr. Hawkins was vice president for assessment programs at the National Board of Medical Examiners (NBME) in Philadelphia, where he helped implement the Clinical Skills Examination of the United States Medical Licensing Examination (USMLE), develop the NBME's assessment of professional behaviors program, and enhance the post-licensure assessment system of the NBME and Federation of State Medical Boards. Before joining the NBME, Dr. Hawkins was Assistant Dean and Director of the Simulation Center at the Uniformed Services University of the Health Sciences. He is board-certified by the American Board of Internal Medicine in internal medicine with a subspecialty in infectious diseases.

Eric S. Holmboe, MD, MACP, FRCP, FAoME (hon)

Eric S. Holmboe, MD, MACP, FRCP, FAoME (hon), is Senior Vice President, Milestones Development and Evaluation at the Accreditation Council for Graduate Medical Education (ACGME). He is also Professor Adjunct of Medicine at Yale University and Adjunct Professor of Medicine at the Uniformed Services University of the Health Sciences and Feinberg School of Medicine at Northwestern University.

He also served as Associate Program Director, Yale Primary Care Internal Medicine Residency Program; Director of Student Clinical Assessment, Yale School of Medicine; and Assistant Director of the Yale Robert Wood Johnson Clinical Scholars program. Before joining Yale in 2000, he served as Division Chief of General Internal Medicine at the National Naval Medical Center. Dr. Holmboe retired from the US Naval Reserves in 2005.

His research interests include interventions to improve quality of care and methods in the assessment of clinical competence. His professional memberships include the American College of Physicians, where he is a Master of the College, Society of General Internal Medicine, and Association of Medical Education in Europe. He is an honorary Fellow of the Royal College of Physicians in London and the Academy of Medical Educators.

Dr. Holmboe is a graduate of Franklin and Marshall College and the University of Rochester School of Medicine. He completed his residency and chief residency at Yale-New Haven Hospital, and was a Robert Wood Johnson Clinical Scholar at Yale University.

Jan Jones-Schenk, DHSc, RN, NE-BC

Jan Jones-Schenk, DHSc, RN, NE-BC, has worked in a variety of clinical nursing and health care leadership roles. She served six years on the Board of Directors of the American Nurses Association and is Past President of the American Nurses Credentialing Center (ANCC). She spearheaded the development of ANCC's international unit (Credentialing International) and has presented widely in Europe and the UK on nursing accreditation and credentialing.

Dr. Jones-Schenk has a master's degree in nursing administration, is a board-certified nurse administrator and has a doctorate in health sciences with an emphasis on global health. She is the 2015 recipient of the US Distance Learning Association's Award for Outstanding Leadership by an Individual in the Field of Distance Learning. She currently serves as National Director for the College of Health Professions for Western Governors University, which offers degrees in nursing, health informatics, and health administration, and has over 20,000 students enrolled nationwide. She serves on the board of MedU, a medical education company, and is the Vice President for Membership for the Council on Graduate Education for Administration in Nursing. She is an associate editor for the monthly leadership column for the *Journal of Continuing Education in Nursing*. Dr. Jones-Schenk is a national expert on competency-based education and learning science.

Adina L. Kalet, MD, MPH

Adina L. Kalet, MD, MPH, Arnold P. Gold Professor of Humanism and Professionalism, has devoted her career to ensuring that public investment in health professionals training leads to improved health outcomes in those they serve. A primary care internist by training, she has appointments in both the departments of Medicine and Surgery and has held a number of leadership positions at the New York University School of Medicine (NYUSOM). Combining her training in both health services and medical education research, she has served as the PI on several grants, including from the NSF and NIH to conduct a seven-institution randomized controlled trial of WISE-MD, and is founding Director of Research for both the Program on Medical Education and Technology (PMET) and the Research on Medical Education Outcomes (ROMEO) initiative, a group of cross-disciplinary researchers dedicated to conducting the education and health services research linking medical education to long-term outcomes in learners and patients. Along with Drs. Sondra Zabar, Colleen Gillespie, and Lisa Altshuler, she leads the Program on Medical Education Innovations and Research (PrMEIR). Dr. Kalet also directs the NYU Clinical Translational Science Institute Translational Research Education and Careers Mentor Development Program (NYU CTSI TREC MDP), which prepares 15–20 researchers annually for their role in mentoring translational research. She runs the Peer Mentor Training for the Programs to Increase Diversity among Individuals Engaged in Health-Related Research (PRIDE) in the NYU Department of Population Health. In 2014, she co-edited a book entitled *Remediation in Medical Education: A Midcourse Correction* (Springer). In 2015, along with Dr. David Stern, she led the collaboration with the University of Maastricht School of Health Professions Education to launch the NYU-Maastricht Masters in Health Professions Education to enhance the capacity for medical educational scholarship in the US. Dr. Kalet and her husband Mark Schwartz (Vice Chair for Education for the Department of Population Health, NYU) met during residency (on BH 16E). They have two children and an evolving number of pets and live happily in Brooklyn, NY.

Debra L. Klamen, MD, MHPE

Debra L. Klamen, MD, MHPE, received her MD in 1985 from the University of Chicago, and did a psychiatry residency at the University of Illinois at Chicago (UIC) from 1985–1989. She then received her master's of health professional education from UIC in 1998. She has attended the Harvard Macy Program for Physician Educators (1995), the Hedwig van Ameringen Executive Leadership in Academic Medicine Program for Women (2001–2002), and the Harvard Macy Program for Leaders in Healthcare Education (2005). After running a general adult inpatient psychiatric unit for five years, Dr. Klamen became the Director of Undergraduate Medical Education in Psychiatry at UIC from 1994–2002. From 1998–2002, she became first the Assistant Dean for Preclerkship Curriculum at UIC, then the Associate Dean for Undergraduate Curriculum, until assuming the position of Senior Associate Dean for Education & Curriculum; Professor and Chair, Department of Medical Education at Southern Illinois University School of Medicine (SIUSOM) in early 2004.

Dr. Klamen has been heavily involved in undergraduate curriculum and assessment innovations for much of her career. Examples include the development of UIC's Essentials of Clinical Medicine course, an active learning, small-group-based course incorporating clinical skills training into the first two years of medical school. She created, developed, and implemented SIUSOM's Longitudinal Performance Examination, a clinical reasoning progress test, which is now used by five medical schools around the country. She designed SIUSOM's senior clinical competency examination remediation course in 2006. Dr. Klamen was responsible for the development of SIUSOM's diagnostic justification exercise, which examines the clinical reasoning skills of students throughout their four years of medical school, and is the subject of this project's work. She headed the innovations curriculum committee at SIUSOM and was at the forefront of the development of the innovative new third-year clerkship curriculum, which began at SIU in July 2016. Dr. Klamen has been active for much of her career in publishing scholarly work in the areas of clinical reasoning, the diagnosis and remediation of students failing standardized patient examinations, and preparation of students to enter residency.

Steven A. Lieberman, MD

Steven A. Lieberman, MD, is Professor in the Department of Internal Medicine, Division of Endocrinology at the University of Texas Medical Branch in Galveston and is currently serving as Interim Dean at the UT Rio Grande Valley School of Medicine. He has served in the Dean's office in Galveston for 16 years in a variety of roles, including curriculum dean, vice dean for academic affairs, and senior dean for administration, overseeing numerous educational programs while pursuing research related to medical education. He has held medical education service and leadership roles within the University of Texas System. In addition, he has worked in numerous capacities with the National Board of Medical Examiners since 2004. A native of San Antonio, he completed his undergraduate degree at Stanford; medical school at UT Southwestern in Dallas; internal medicine residency in San Jose, California; and endocrinology fellowship at Stanford. After brief service on the faculty of the George Washington University School of Medicine faculty, he returned to Texas in 1994 to join the faculty at UTMB.

Kimberly D. Lomis, MD

Kimberly D. Lomis, MD, is Associate Dean for Undergraduate Medical Education, Professor of Surgery, and Professor of Medical Education and Administration at Vanderbilt University School of Medicine. She was charged with the implementation of a major revision of the medical school curriculum, "Curriculum 2.0." Dr. Lomis also serves in the AAMC as the Associate Project Director for the national pilot of the Core EPAs for Entering Residency, and she is the past-chair of the Section on

Undergraduate Medical Education of the Group on Educational Affairs. In the AMA Accelerating Change in Medical Education consortium, Dr. Lomis is a PI and co-leader of the competency-based assessment group.

Dr. Lomis received her BS from the University of Texas at Austin in 1988 and her MD from the University Texas Southwestern Medical School in 1992. She trained in general surgery at Vanderbilt University Medical Center from 1992–1997 and practiced until 2012. She holds a graduate certificate in the Business of Medicine from Johns Hopkins, and is a Harvard Macy Institute Scholar.

Dr. Lomis' academic interests include complex systems, change management, and competency-based medical education. She guided the implementation of competency milestones for UME at Vanderbilt, which served as evidence of student development in the new digital portfolio. She is invested in program evaluation and promoting the judicial use of educational resources.

Catherine R. Lucey, MD

Catherine R. Lucey, MD, a board-certified internist, is Executive Vice Dean, Vice Dean for Education, Professor of Medicine, and holder of the Faustino and Martha Molina Bernadett Presidential Chair in Medical Education at the University of California, San Francisco (UCSF) School of Medicine. Previously, she was the Interim Dean, College of Medicine, Vice Dean for Education at The Ohio State University (OSU) College of Medicine. A past chair of the Board of Directors of the American Board of Internal Medicine, she currently serves on the Board of Directors of the Association of Academic Medical Centers and the American Board of Medical Specialties. She is Chair of the AAMC MCAT Validity Study.

Dr. Lucey was a Clinical Instructor at Harvard University School of Medicine, Assistant Professor of Medicine at the University of Texas Health Sciences Center at San Antonio, and Associate Professor of Medicine at the George Washington University School of Medicine and the Uniformed Services University of the Health Sciences, before joining The Ohio State University as Associate Professor of Medicine in 2002. She was promoted to Professor of Internal Medicine in 2005. She has won numerous teaching awards and has given hundreds of invited presentations at national meetings and academic institutions across the country. Her areas of expertise include professionalism, curricular redesign and leadership. Her 2011 *JAMA* Internal Medicine paper "Medical Education: Part of the Problem and Part of the Solution" proposed a new vision of the physician competencies needed for 21st century medical practice. The UCSF Bridges Curriculum embeds these competencies in a novel framework of authentic workplace learning and scientific discovery experiences. Dr. Lucey is a co-author of the book *Understanding Medical Professionalism* (McGraw Hill), released in 2014.

A Fellow of the American College of Physicians, Dr. Lucey is a prior council member for both the Society of General Internal Medicine and the Association of Program Directors in Internal Medicine. She served on the AAMC MR5 Committee, charged with redesigning the MCAT.

Dr. Lucey earned her medical degree from the Northwestern University School of Medicine, and completed her residency in internal medicine at UCSF before serving as chief resident in internal medicine at the San Francisco General Hospital.

Dylan Masters, MD

Dylan Masters, MD, is a resident physician in Anesthesia at the University of California, San Francisco (UCSF). He enjoys practicing medicine at the many different UCSF-affiliated hospitals in the San Francisco Bay Area. He is currently in intern year, rotating through a variety of disciplines, and will settle down with Anesthesia starting in July 2017 as a CA-1. He is one of UCSF's Critical Care Scholars, and will stay on an extra year for an integrated fellowship in Critical Care.

He is passionate about education and enjoys exploring it at work, through research, and when not in the hospital. He has been a teacher at heart since growing up in the San Francisco Bay Area, and started out teaching on the museum floor at the California Academy of Sciences. He tutored physics and taught outdoor education in Maine at Bowdoin College. Before medical school, he taught physics and math in the Peace Corps in Tanzania for two years. During medical school at UCSF, he led education outreach programs for the first few years, and led many first-year small groups in his fourth year.

Otherwise, you can find him outside hiking or playing tennis, or in the kitchen cooking up something new. Ask him about his favorite recipes or his thoughts on how to best cook a turkey!

George C. Mejicano, MD, MS, FACP, FACEHP

George C. Mejicano, MD, MS, FACP, FACEHP, received his medical degree from the University of Illinois and completed his post-graduate training at the University of Wisconsin. He is board-certified in both internal medicine and adult infectious diseases and is actively participating and meeting all requirements stipulated by the ABIM regarding Maintenance of Certification. He is Professor of Medicine in the Division of Infectious Diseases at Oregon Health & Science University (OHSU). His clinical interests include travel medicine, antibiotic resistance, and emerging infections. Dr. Mejicano has served on the Board of Scientific Counselors of the National Center for Infectious Diseases at the CDC and was Interim Head of the Section of Infectious Diseases at the University of Wisconsin School of Medicine and Public Health from 2007–2008.

In addition to his clinical qualifications, Dr. Mejicano has a master's degree in adult education from the University of Wisconsin. His educational interests include competency-based medical education and outcomes assessment. He has done research on how education can lead to improvements in medical practice and was awarded the Felch Award for Research in Continuing Medical Education by the Alliance for CME in 2002. He currently serves as the Senior Associate Dean for Education at OHSU where he oversees the entire educational portfolio—UME, GME, CME/CPD, graduate studies and faculty development—for the School of Medicine. He is the leader of OHSU's team working on the AAMC's pilot program studying the 13 Core Entrustable Professional Activities for Entering Residency and is the PI of a five-year, $1 million grant from the AMA's Accelerating Change in Medical Education strategic initiative.

Dr. Mejicano has served on the Board of Directors of the ACCME and is the recipient of the Bob Razkowski "Hero Award" from that organization. In addition, he has served as a consultant for the ABMS regarding Maintenance of Certification and served as President of the Alliance for Continuing Education in the Health Professions. He is Chair-Elect of the AMA's Academic Physicians Section and also serves as Chair of the Continuing Education and Improvement Section of the AAMC's Group on Educational Affairs. He has received numerous teaching awards from students, residents, and faculty peers, and he is a sought-after speaker who has given hundreds of national and international presentations during his career.

Richard K. Reznick, MD, MEd, FRCSC, FACS, FRCSEd (hon), FRCSI (hon)

Richard K. Reznick, MD, MEd, FRCSC, FACS, FRCSEd (hon), FRCSI (hon), is married to Cheryl, and they have three children—Joanna, Josh and Gabe. Born in Montreal, he received his undergraduate university education and medical degree from McGill University, followed by a general surgical residency at the University of Toronto. He spent two years in fellowship training, first obtaining a master's degree in medical education from Southern Illinois University, followed by a fellowship in colorectal surgery at the University of Texas in Houston.

Since his first faculty appointment at the University of Toronto in 1987, Dr. Reznick has been active in both colorectal surgery and research in medical education. He was instrumental in developing a performance-based examination, which is now used for medical licensure in Canada. He ran a research program on assessment of technical competence for surgeons and supervised a fellowship program in surgical education.

At the University of Toronto Faculty of Medicine, he was the inaugural Director of the Faculty's Centre for Research in Education at University Health Network (The Wilson Centre) from 1997 to 2002. In 1999, he was appointed Vice President of Education at University Health Network. He served eight years as the R. S. McLaughlin Professor and Chairman of the Department of Surgery at the University of Toronto from 2002–2010.

In July 2010, Dr. Reznick assumed the position of Dean, Faculty of Health Sciences at Queen's University and Chief Executive Officer of the Southeastern Ontario Academic Medical Organization (SEAMO).

Dr. Reznick has received numerous awards for his work in education, including the Royal College of Physicians and Surgeons of Canada Medal in Surgery and the James H. Graham Award of Merit, the Association for Surgical Education Distinguished Educator Award, the National Board of Medical Examiners John P. Hubbard Award, the Daniel C. Tosteson Award for Leadership in Medical Education, the 2006 Inaugural University of Toronto President's Teaching Award and the Karolinska Institutet Prize for Research in Medical Education. In 2015, he was the recipient of McGill University's Medicine Alumni Global Award for Lifetime Achievement. Dr. Reznick is a honourary fellow of the Royal College of Surgeons of Edinburgh and the Royal College of Surgeons of Ireland.

Dr. Reznick is the author of over 130 peer-reviewed publications and has delivered nearly 300 lectures to hospitals, universities, and scientific organizations around the world.

Denise V. Rodgers, MD, FAAFP

Denise V. Rodgers, MD, FAAFP, is Vice Chancellor for Interprofessional Programs at Rutgers Biomedical and Health Sciences. She is also the Hunterdon Chair in Interprofessional Education at Rutgers-Robert Wood Johnson Medical School where she is a professor in the Department of Family Medicine and Community Health. Prior to these appointments, Dr. Rodgers served as the fifth and final president of the University of Medicine and Dentistry of New Jersey (UMDNJ) from January 1, 2012, to June 30, 2013. From April 2006 to June 2013, Dr. Rodgers led UMDNJ's academic and clinical operations as Executive Vice President. She served as UMDNJ Chief of Staff from 2005 to 2006. From 1997 to 2005, Dr. Rodgers was Senior Associate Dean for Community Health at the UMDNJ-Robert Wood Johnson Medical School.

Prior to joining UMDNJ, Dr. Rodgers was professor and vice chair in the University of California, San Francisco Department of Family and Community Medicine and director of the San Francisco General Hospital (SFGH) Family Medicine Residency Program. She also served as Family Medicine Chief of Service at SFGH. From 1994 to 1996 she served as Chief of Staff at SFGH.

Dr. Rodgers received a Bachelor of Arts in psychobiology from Oberlin College and graduated from Michigan State University College of Human Medicine. She completed her family medicine training in the Residency Program in Social Medicine at Montefiore Medical Center in the Bronx.

Dr. Rodgers is board-certified in family medicine and is a diplomate of the American Academy of Family Physicians.

Stephen C. Schoenbaum, MD, MPH

Stephen C. Schoenbaum, MD, MPH, is Special Advisor to the President of the Josiah Macy Jr. Foundation. He has extensive experience as a clinician, epidemiologist, and manager. From 2000–2010, he was Executive Vice President for Programs at The Commonwealth Fund and Executive Director of its Commission on High Performance Health Systems. Prior to that, he was Medical Director and then President of Harvard Pilgrim Health Care of New England, a mixed-model HMO delivery system in Providence, RI.

He is an adjunct professor of healthcare leadership at Brown University; a founder of what is now the Department of Population Medicine at Harvard Medical School (formerly the Department of Ambulatory Care and Prevention); author of over 175 professional publications; the chair of the International Advisory Committee to the Joyce and Irving Goldman Medical School, Ben Gurion University, Beer Sheva, Israel; and an honorary fellow of the Royal College of Physicians.

Daniel Schumacher, MD, MEd

Daniel Schumacher, MD, MEd, is an assistant professor in the division of Emergency Medicine at Cincinnati Children's, where he chairs the education research focus group.

Dan is a member of the Pediatrics Milestone Project Working Group, which has led him to publish and lecture widely on the Milestone Project, both within and outside the pediatric community.

A former associate program director and director of competency-based assessment for one of the premier pediatric residencies in the country, Dan brings practical experience to his current research-focused roles. The bulk of his current research focuses in three main areas. First, he is conducting a series of studies as part of a PhD program that seek to understand the association between entrustment decisions and indicators of quality care. Second, he is the co-PI for a national study of the general pediatrics entrustable professional activities that have been developed by The American Board of Pediatrics. Finally, he recently completed data collection as the PI for a national study looking at how clinical competency committees (CCC) function and make decisions, as well as the association between milestone assignments made by CCC members and program directors and recommended advancement decisions these individuals also make.

Dr. Schumacher has been a Visiting Scholar of The American Board of Pediatrics and the American Board of Medical Specialties. He has been part of national efforts of The American Board of Pediatrics, Accreditation Council for Graduate Medical Education, Association of American Medical Colleges, National Board of Medical Examiners, Federation of Pediatric Organizations, American Academy of Pediatrics, Association of Pediatric Program Directors, and Academic Pediatric Association.

Juliann G. Sebastian, PhD, RN, FAAN

Juliann G. Sebastian, PhD, RN, FAAN, was appointed Dean and Professor of the University of Nebraska Medical Center, College of Nursing in October, 2011. She previously served as Dean of the College of Nursing at the University of Missouri-St. Louis and earlier as Assistant Dean for Advanced Practice Nursing and Professor at the University of Kentucky, College of Nursing. Dr. Sebastian earned her bachelor and master of science in nursing from the University of Kentucky, College of Nursing, and her doctorate in business administration from the University of Kentucky College of Business and Economics.

Her areas of expertise are organization of care delivery systems, community-based care for underserved populations, academic nursing practice, and Doctor of Nursing Practice curricula.

She has been actively engaged in shaping national academic nursing policies through her service on many task forces for the American Association of Colleges of Nursing (AACN) and as an AACN Board Member. She currently serves as Chair of the Board of Directors for AACN (2016–2018) and recently completed a term as Chair of the Board of the Global Alliance for Leadership in Nursing Education and Science (2015–2017).

Olle (Th.J.) ten Cate, PhD

Olle (Th.J.) ten Cate, PhD, attended medical school at the University of Amsterdam, the Netherlands, and has spent his professional life, from 1980 on, serving medical education. In 1986, he completed a PhD dissertation on peer teaching in medical education. Until 1999, he was closely involved with all the University of Amsterdam's major preclinical and clinical curriculum reforms, education research, program evaluation, and educational development. In 1999, he was appointed full professor of Medical Education at Utrecht University, the Netherlands, and program director of undergraduate medical education at University Medical Center Utrecht (UMCU). Since 2005, he has led the Center for Research and Development of Education at UMCU. His research interests include curriculum development, peer teaching, competency-based medical education, and many other topics. From 2006 until 2012 he served as president of the Netherlands Association for Medical Education. In 2012, he was appointed adjunct professor of medicine at the University of California, San Francisco, next to his work in Utrecht, to execute a collaborative doctoral program in health professions education. He has published extensively in the medical education literature (250+) and supervised and supervises many doctoral students (25+) in health professions education research. He serves on the editorial boards of *Medical Teacher* and the *Journal of Graduate Medical Education*, and is a Fellow and member of the Executive Committee of the Association for Medical Education in Europe. In 2017, he received the John P. Hubbard Award of the US National Board of Medical Examiners.

George E. Thibault, MD

George E. Thibault, MD became the seventh president of the Josiah Macy Jr. Foundation in January 2008. Immediately prior to that, he served as Vice President of Clinical Affairs at Partners Healthcare System in Boston and Director of the Academy at Harvard Medical School (HMS). He was the first Daniel D. Federman Professor of Medicine and Medical Education at HMS and is now the Federman Professor, Emeritus.

Dr. Thibault previously served as Chief Medical Officer at Brigham and Women's Hospital and as Chief of Medicine at the Harvard-affiliated Brockton/West Roxbury VA Hospital. He was Associate Chief of Medicine and Director of the Internal Medical Residency Program at the Massachusetts General Hospital (MGH). At the MGH he also served as Director of the Medical ICU and the Founding Director of the Medical Practice Evaluation Unit.

For nearly four decades at HMS, Dr. Thibault played leadership roles in many aspects of undergraduate and graduate medical education. He played a central role in the New Pathway Curriculum reform and was a leader in the new Integrated Curriculum reform at HMS. He was the Founding Director of the Academy at HMS, which was created to recognize outstanding teachers and to promote innovations in medical education. Throughout his career he has been recognized for his roles in teaching and mentoring medical students, residents, fellows and junior faculty. In addition to his teaching, his research has focused on the evaluation of practices and outcomes of medical intensive care and variations in the use of cardiac technologies.

Dr. Thibault is Chairman of the Board of the MGH Institute of Health Professions, Chairman of the Board of the New York Academy of Medicine, and he serves on the Boards of the Institute on Medicine as a Profession and the Arnold P. Gold Foundation. He served on the President's White House Fellows Commission during the Obama Administration and for twelve years he chaired the Special Medical

Advisory Group for the Department of Veterans Affairs. He is past President of the Harvard Medical Alumni Association and Past Chair of Alumni Relations at HMS. He is a member of the National Academy of Medicine.

Dr. Thibault graduated summa cum laude from Georgetown University in 1965 and magna cum laude from Harvard Medical School in 1969. He completed his internship and residency in medicine and fellowship in cardiology at Massachusetts General Hospital. He also trained in cardiology at the National Heart and Lung Institute in Bethesda and at Guys Hospital in London, and served as Chief Resident in Medicine at MGH.

Dr. Thibault has been the recipient of numerous awards and honors from Georgetown (Ryan Prize in Philosophy, Alumni Prize, and Cohongaroton Speaker) and Harvard (Alpha Omega Alpha, Henry Asbury Christian Award and Society of Fellows). He has been a visiting Scholar both at the Institute of Medicine and Harvard's Kennedy School of Government and a Visiting Professor of Medicine at numerous medical schools in the U.S. and abroad. In 2017 he was the recipient of the Abraham Flexner Award for Distinguished Service to Medical Education from the Association of American Medical Colleges and he was made an honorary Fellow of the American Academy of Nursing. He has received honorary doctoral degrees from Georgetown University, Wake Forest University and The Commonwealth Medical College.

Peter H. Vlasses, PharmD, DSc (Hon.), FCCP

Peter H. Vlasses, PharmD, DSc (Hon.), FCCP, received his Bachelor of Science and Doctor of Pharmacy degrees from the Philadelphia College of Pharmacy and Science (PCPS) and served a residency in hospital pharmacy at Thomas Jefferson University Hospital in Philadelphia, PA. His professional experience includes service as a clinical faculty member at The Ohio State University College of Pharmacy and PCPS. He served as Head of the Clinical Research Unit and Research Associate Professor of Medicine and Pharmacology, Jefferson Medical College, in Philadelphia, and then as Associate Director, Clinical Practice Advancement Center, and Director, Clinical Research & Investigator Services, University HealthSystem Consortium, Oak Brook, Illinois. Dr. Vlasses is a Founding Member, Fellow, and Past-President of the American College of Clinical Pharmacy (ACCP) and was a board-certified pharmacotherapy specialist from 1994 to 2016. He served on the Board of Directors of the Association of Specialized and Professional Accreditors (ASPA), as Chair and Treasurer. He serves on advisory councils for the National Center for Interprofessional Practice and Education, and the O'Neil Center Get Well Network. His awards include the Russell R. Miller Award from ACCP, in recognition of his sustained and outstanding contributions to the biomedical literature; the ASPA Cynthia Davenport Award to recognize exceptional effort on behalf of specialized and professional accreditors; and an Honorary Doctor of Science degree from Mercer University, Atlanta, Georgia.

ACPE is the US agency responsible for the accreditation of professional degree programs in pharmacy and providers of continuing pharmacy education and the evaluation and certification of professional degree programs internationally.

Diane B. Wayne, MD

Diane B. Wayne, MD, is Vice Dean for Education and the Dr. John Sherman Appleman Professor of Medicine at the Northwestern University Feinberg School of Medicine. She is also Chair of the Department of Medical Education and President of the McGaw Medical Center of Northwestern University. Dr. Wayne has received many honors and awards, including the 2016 Mentor of the Year award from the medical school, the 2015 Patterson Award, bestowed annually by the graduating resident class to the Best Teacher in the Department of Medicine, and the 2014 Leader in General Internal Medicine Award from the Society of General Internal Medicine, Midwest Region. Dr. Wayne has been invited to deliver numerous talks and lectures and has served as a visiting professor at many national and international institutions and conferences. Dr. Wayne received her bachelor's and medical degrees from Northwestern University and completed her residency at University of Chicago Hospitals. Following a faculty appointment at Baylor College of Medicine in Houston, Texas, she has since 2001 served as faculty in the Department of Medicine and since 2009 in the Department of Medical Education for the Northwestern University Feinberg School of Medicine. She was named Vice Dean for Education in 2014.

As a researcher, Dr. Wayne focuses on the intersection of education and patient care quality. Her expertise is in simulation-based research. Her team has shown that high-quality education leads to improved clinical skills, reduced iatrogenic complications, and lower hospital costs than traditional approaches. She has published extensively on these topics in notable peer-reviewed journals such as *Academic Medicine*, the *American Journal of Medical Quality*, the *Archives of Internal Medicine*, *Critical Care Medicine*, and *CHEST*.

Alison J. Whelan, MD

Alison J. Whelan, MD, chief medical education officer, leads AAMC initiatives to transform the current models of education and workforce preparation across the full continuum of medical education. She also directs AAMC efforts that support medical education officers, regional campuses, education researchers, students, and residents.

Prior to joining the association in 2016, Dr. Whelan had been a member of the faculty at Washington University School of Medicine since 1994. In 1997, she was appointed associate dean for medical student education and in 2009 was appointed senior associate dean for education. During her tenure, Dr. Whelan coordinated the creation of the Practice of Medicine curriculum and led the planning for the school's new education building and the creation of the Center for Interprofessional Education.

Dr. Whelan received her bachelor's degree from Carleton College in 1981. She earned her medical degree from Washington University in 1986 and completed her postgraduate work and residency at the former Barnes Hospital, now Barnes-Jewish Hospital.

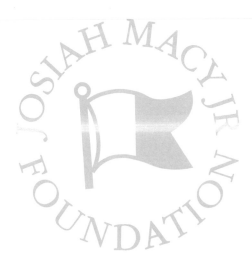

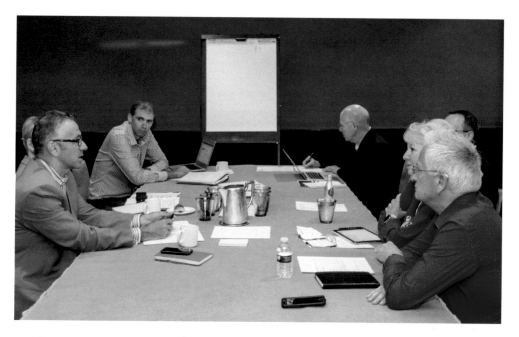

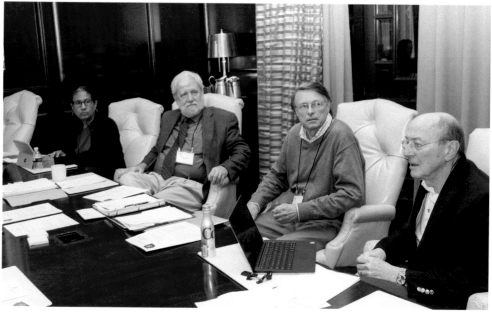

Copy Editor: Jesse Y. Jou
Production Editor: Yasmine R. Legendre
Designed by: Vixjo Design, Inc.
Photos by: Jared Gruenwald Photography

ISBN# 978-0-914362-34-0

Printed in U.S.A. with soy-based inks on paper containing post-consumer
recycled content and produced using 100% wind-generated power

Josiah Macy Jr. Foundation
44 East 64th Street, New York, NY 10065 www.macyfoundation.org